Policy Innovation for Health

Ilona Kickbusch
Editor

Policy Innovation for Health

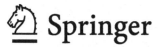 Springer

Editor
Ilona Kickbusch
Graduate Institute of International
   and Developmental Studies
Geneva
Switzerland
kickbusch@bluewin.ch
ilona.kickbusch@graduateinstitute.ch

ISBN: 978-1-4419-2730-9   e-ISBN: 978-0-387-79876-9
DOI 10.1007/978-0-387-79876-9

Printed on acid-free paper

springer.com

Acknowledgements

This book is the result of a 2-year conversation between the six authors during the period 2006–2008. We were able to have a number of in-depth discussion meetings and engage in a challenging intellectual debate and exchange – a situation rarely available in the hectic life of modern academia. We were also able to test our thinking during this period by giving talks and lectures at major conferences, inviting policy makers and innovators and putting our ideas to the test with our local collaborators and colleagues. For an editor it was a special privilege to be so fully involved with such a distinguished group of colleagues. This approach to producing the book was made possible through the support of Merck & Co. Inc., Whitehouse Station, NJ, USA* as all authors of this book are members of the MSD Academic Advisory Board on Health Policy Innovation.

The mission developed by the group was twofold: to explore and map policy innovations in health governance in OECD countries and to cultivate relationships and stimulate discussion with other institutions and among key leaders and decision makers. The aim was to do this through knowledge production, constructive conversations, and policy learning and transfer. This has been achieved in many ways – and will culminate in the presentation of this book at the 2008 EUPHA European Public Health Association Conference in Lisbon, Portugal, which will focus on "I-Health: health and innovation in Europe."

As members of the advisory board we would like to thank the two members of Merck & Co. who worked with us through this period: Jeffrey Sturchio and Melinda Hanisch. Their support and patience as we grappled with difficult intellectual concepts was much appreciated, as was their input to our discussion. We would also like to acknowledge the intellectual work that was produced by the Academic Advisory Board – chaired by Marshall Marinker – in the years before our own work – we drew heavily from the effort of those earlier years – in particular the work on health targets and health values.

We hope the readers will find this book as stimulating as we experienced our time working together.

Brienz, Switzerland   Ilona Kickbusch

---

*Merck & Co., Inc., Whitehouse Station, NJ, USA operates in most countries outside North America as Merck, Sharp & Dohme, or MSD.

Contents

Chapter 1
Policy Innovations for Health

Ilona Kickbusch

Abstract We are at a turning point in health policy. It has become increasingly clear that changes in the existing health care system will not be sufficient to maintain and improve our health at this historical juncture. Both our extensive knowledge on what creates health as well as the exponentially rising rates of chronic disease, obesity, and mental health problems indicate that we need to shift course and apply a radically new mind-set to health and health policy. This is what we mean by policy innovations for health. The boundaries of what we call the "health system" are becoming increasingly fluid and health has become integral to how we live our everyday life. Health itself has become a major economic and social driving force in society. This shifts the pressure for policy innovation from a focus on the existing health system to a reorganization of how we approach health in 21st century societies. The dynamics of the health society challenge the way we conceptualize and locate health in the policy arena and the mechanisms through which we conduct health policy. They also redefine who should be involved in the policy process. This concern is beginning to be addressed within government through Health in All Policy approaches and beyond government through new partnerships for health. Most importantly, the role of citizen and patient is being redefined – a development that will probably lead to the most significant of the policy innovations for health in the 21st century.

Introduction

> *Innovation is something everyone wants more of, but no-*
> *body is too sure what it means exactly.* John Gapper [1]

Innovation for the authors of this book is about applying a radically new mindset to health and health policy with the goal of addressing the determinants of health and involving citizens in their health in new ways. This explains our choice of terminology: policy innovations *for* health. We start from a perspective that considers

I. Kickbusch (✉)
The Graduate Institute Geneva, PO Box 136, CH 1211 Geneva 21, Switzerland
kickbusch@bluewin.ch, ilona.kickbusch@graduateinstitute.ch

I. Kickbusch (ed.), *Policy Innovation for Health*,
DOI 10.1007/978-0-387-79876-9_1, © Springer Science+Business Media, LLC 2009

both health and innovation to be central driving forces in 21st century societies, and we maintain that their prominent role reflects major societal shifts that are under way. The consequence is not only a changing role of health in modern societies but also a new perception of innovation in relation to health.

As part of this change we see new mechanisms emerge which aim to address the seminal changes underway in health and society. The shift from the industrial society of the 19th and 20th centuries to the knowledge societies of the 21st century is as ground-breaking as was the shift from the agrarian to the industrial world – and they are similar in their deep impact on health, this increases the need for innovation. The changes in our way of life are shaping our lifestyles and have created a situation where many of the patterns of everyday life – for example, our eating and food shopping patterns – and new forms of social stratification – for example, new forms of social inclusion and exclusion – endanger our health. This means that we need to understand that the health challenges and the diseases that come with this change are of a larger societal, not an individual nature.

It seems obvious that this development has two consequences: it changes the role of the health care sector significantly toward managing chronic disease rather than acute care and it moves many of the solutions for the most challenging health problems into other social and policy arenas. The authors of this book are focused on the second challenge and the policy mechanisms that are needed to address it. The need for change is vast. First, there is hardly a policy sector that can be excluded: health, education, agriculture, transport, industry, consumer affairs, and sports – all are essential to support health. Second, in a consumer society the role of business is critical and consumers themselves must express their demand. Finally, communities must act for their health interest and individuals are required to support their individual health and that of their families in new ways. To do so they need to be able to negotiate and navigate an increasingly complex health and care environment.

A recent analysis concerned with innovation and high performing health systems [2] underlines that there are two goals of innovation in relation to health: improving the affordability, quality, and efficiency of the health care system and improving the health of populations. Ideally the two would be fully complementary – in the real world they are not. Usually when we speak of innovation in the context of health the automatic assumption is that we mean the expansion of therapeutic possibilities – we associate new medicines, new technologies, and increasingly the potential of biomedicine and genetics. Sometimes we think of new approaches to the organization and financing of the medical care system, then we typically speak of "health care reform" – a term that is now linked almost exclusively with efficiency, effectiveness, and cost saving. The words innovation and health policy do not by and large sit very well together because the notion of "newness" and "better" that is at the core of innovation has been overshadowed by many short-term reorganizations of health care systems that seem to lack in vision and long-term perspective. And, if innovation is considered in terms of radical innovation only then we experience a clear tension between the drive for innovation and the constant challenge to keep down health care expenditures. A recent Health Innovation Survey by the OECD [3] typically focuses on the "question how to encourage and foster innovation which addresses health needs and priorities, maximizes access to benefits, and manages challenges and risks in a way that is beneficial to both innovators and health systems." Innovation in this case is also mainly related to innovations in biotechnology and the key challenge is how OECD countries are able to cope with introducing such technical and product-based innovations into their respective health care systems. This focus on financial pressure has led – through a range of new assessment mechanisms – to a reinforcement of a binary understanding of innovation as being either radical or incremental and a focus on medical rather than social value.

The Shift to the Health Society

Over the last decade we have begun to witness a major shift with regard to health and its role in society. I argue that we now live in a *health society* which is characterized by two major social processes: *the expansion of the territory of health* and *the expansion of the reflectivity of health* [4]. The creation of the health society of the 21st century has been a process long in the making, beginning from about the mid 17th century onward. Health is integral to modernity and our modern societies would not be possible without the health gains achieved in this 250-year period [5]. During this time the balance of power between the four domains of the health system – *personal health, public health, medical health,* and *the health market* – has shifted continuously. The domains of personal health and public health dominated the 18th and 19th centuries, while during the 20th century the medical health domain gained increasing strength both in terms of its power over the social definition of health and the dominance of its organizational and governance infrastructure; this process of dominance has been referred to as medicalization. As a consequence, in both political and public perceptions, the social organization of health resides in what we have come to call the health care system and concerns over how to ensure the long-term financial sustainability of this system dominate the health policy debate.

But today the boundaries of what we call the "health care system" are becoming increasingly fluid. Health has become integral to how we live our everyday life. In this health is similar to innovation, which is also increasingly defined as being fluid, an issue that will be reflected upon later in this chapter. Indeed the expansion and liquidity of boundaries is a major characteristic of what the sociologist Zygmunt Bauman calls "liquid modernity" [6]. This changes the health policy debate because it means that *health is everywhere*: every policy decision a government makes also impacts on health and at the individual level every behavioral choice also has a health consequence. This was always the case – but now it is part of reflective modernity. Most discussions on health policy do not yet take this deep seminal change into account – they still focus on tinkering with a well-defined functional system of health governance, where through a process of defining the evidence base, they aim to ensure clear boundaries, define interventions, and prioritize medical rather than social solutions. The authors of this book are of the opinion that we clearly need a policy approach that responds more adequately to the new environment of 21st century health.

The dynamics of the health society not only challenge the way we conceptualize and locate health and how we conduct health policy but they also redefine who should be involved in policy making – together they constitute policy innovations for health. The chapters of the book further explore five key defining concepts:

1. health is more than disease and health outcomes need to be measured differently;
2. the system boundaries are shifting and organization of health in society is increasingly separated from the management of disease and illness;
3. health policy is more than health care policy and becomes a joined up process of Health in All Policies at all levels of governance;
4. the differentiation into a first and second health market is occurring rapidly and we are faced with new issues of financing both health and health care;
5. people themselves are major actors in the health arena and new technologies are allowing them to participate in completely new ways.

Many analysts make the point that the changes facing the health sector will be as phenomenal as those we have witnessed in information technology and communications. This is due to the fact that health itself has become a major economic and social driving force in society [7] and that good health outcomes are increasingly important for a range of societal goals. The Conference Board of Canada [2]suggests understanding innovation "as a means by which societies, systems or organizations achieve social or economic value (e.g. increasing positive health outcomes)"; they maintain that innovation occurs only when new value is created. Our focus in this book is to explore what kind of policy innovations for health are required to achieve better population health, in terms of both its social and economic value. We argue though that the issue at stake is not just another reorganization/improvement of the health care system or a better mechanism of integrating scientific progress into existing heath care systems but a *reorganization of how we approach health in 21st century societies*. In this we follow Peter Drucker's understanding of innovation as creating a new dimension of performance [8].

Conceptualizing Health and Well-Being

In modern democracies health is considered a right. Its doability is driven by the perception that *health* can be created, managed, and produced: *more health is always possible.* It is one of the characteristics of the health society that the notion of *doability* has expanded beyond the ever-rising expectations toward the curative medical care system to impact the determinants of health.

Determinants of Health

The first conceptual starting point for the arguments in this book are the rapidly changing determinants of health. We build on the arguments for increasing the investment for health and well-being and for strengthening the connection between health and wealth which are beginning to be expressed far beyond the public health community. Witness the similarity of the statements from the public health perspective as voiced by Wilkinson and Marmot [9], two of the most respected researchers on social determinants of health

> *Good health involves reducing levels of educational failure, reducing insecurity and unemployment and improving housing standards. Societies that enable all citizens to play a full and useful role in the social, economic and cultural life of their society will be healthier than those where people face insecurity, exclusion and deprivation*

and as expressed in a recent publication commissioned by the European Commission [10]

> *...improving the health status of a population can be beneficial for economic outcomes at the individual and the national level. There is indeed much evidence to suggest that the association between economic wealth and health does not run solely from the former to the latter. An immediate, if general, policy implication that derives from this conclusion is that policy-makers who are interested in improving economic outcomes (e.g. on the labour market or for the entire economy) would have good reasons to consider investment in health as one of their options by which to meet their economic objectives.*

It follows that if societies are to prepare adequately for new health challenges – such as obesity – and if they are to take action on the changes already under way, they must completely rethink their approach to health policy. It is argued that health sustainability is as important as environmental sustainability and that our response must be understood to be the challenge of at least a generation [11]. We need policy innovations for health that address the classic determinants of health, such as education, work, housing, transport, and particularly equity. Some countries – such as Sweden – have now done so and this is discussed in more detail in the chapters that follow [12].

Box 1

The "classic" determinants of health continue to influence our health. They include:

    Income and social status
    Social support networks
    Education and literacy, e.g., health literacy
    Employment/Working conditions
    Social environments/physical environments
    Personal health practices and coping skills
    Healthy child development
    Biology and genetic endowment
    Health services
    Gender
    Culture

(compiled by the Public Health Agency of Canada) [13].

Box 2
Map of the Health and Wellbeing System

The determinants of health

Wellbeing Project
Scotland 2006

However, in the boundaryless health landscape of the 21st century policy innovations are called for that respond to the 21st century determinants of health. Health is increasingly being shaped by forces such as the speed of modern societies, globalization of markets, the increasing mobility and insecurity of individuals, energy expenditure, and concerns regarding risk and safety, and the reach of the media. These forces cut across many of the acknowledged social, environmental, and economic determinants of health. An approach to visualize the many determinants and their interaction was developed by the Well-being Project, Scotland, in a joint effort with members of the community [14].

Understanding of Health

The second conceptual starting point for the authors of this book is an understanding of health which is social rather than a medical. Health governance is now challenged by this conceptualization of health as "well being beyond the absence of disease" as first defined by the World Health Organization in its constitution [15]. The Ottawa Charter of the WHO [16] stated that "health is created in the context of everyday life – where people live, love, work, learn and play," and this has found its expression in a wealth of health promotion activities at organizational, community, and local level. The most well known are the many "settings projects," which aim to create supportive environments for health and encourage people to participate in shaping these settings for everyday life, examples include Healthy Cities, health-promoting schools, and healthy workplaces [17]. Indeed they constitute social innovations that spread the new understanding of health into many different sectors and, as an activity in the space between the sectors, prepare the ground for policy innovations and their social acceptance [18].

Recent global happiness surveys have identified health next to wealth and education as one of the three key factors for societal well-being [19]. Health becomes more central for the aspiration of personal goals in life and social inequalities are increasingly measured in health terms, highlighting differences in health and life expectancy. This broader view of health also needs to be reflected in the way we measure the impact of policy innovation for health. Hernandez-Aguada, in his chapter, discusses the increasing relevance of new types of health intelligence for intersectoral health governance with a particular focus on transparency and accountability for all actors in society. One such example of measurement, The Canadian Index of Well-being [20], clearly illustrates the dimensions of innovation that a new type of health policy needs to address:

- *build a foundation to articulate a shared vision of what really constitutes sustainable well-being;*
- *measure national progress toward, or movement away from, achieving that vision;*
- *understand and promote awareness of why society is moving in the direction it is moving;*
- *stimulate discussion about the types of policies, programs, and activities that would move us closer and faster toward achieving well-being;*
- *give Canadians tools to promote well-being with policy shapers and decision makers;*
- *inform policy by helping policy shapers and decision makers to understand the consequences of their actions for Canadian well-being;*
- *empower Canadians to compare their well-being both with others within Canada and those around the world; and,*
- *add momentum to the global movement for a more holistic way of measuring societal progress.*

Policies must come to terms with the new forces that act to create or compromise health – they must respond to what has been called "the new personal health ecology" where the individuals are subject to a broad range of influences over which they have very little control [21]. Just as cholera was symptomatic for all the dimensions of the rapid urbanization of the 19th century, obesity is the symbolic disease of our global consumer society. It will be a test case for the health governance of the 21st century as was the introduction of water and sewage systems at the end of the 19th century. Such challenges can only be resolved through great political commitment, willingness to innovate, and social action – including social entrepreneurship – at all levels of society.

Locating the Interface Between Innovation and Health

Health and innovation are both social constructs, defined by their time and context. Just as the concept of health is changing, so is the concept of innovation. The social sciences began in the 1970s to concern themselves with both health and innovation as distinct areas of social analysis. It was at this point that both medical sociology (later to become health and medical sociology) and the sociology of innovation began to advance – the one never far removed from medicine, the other never far from the sociological analysis of technological development. Even today much of the literature on innovation still comes from a science and technology perspective. This is in sharp contrast to economics, where already at the beginning of the 20th century Josef Schumpeter drew attention to innovation as the engine of social and economic development, highlighting both its power of creation and of destruction [22].

Health has now become such an innovation engine – many investors see health as "the next big thing" and a rapidly growing health market attaches the added value "health" and well-being to an ever-growing set of products and services. The chapter by Henke and Martin in this book illustrates this process: not only do health innovations change society, but through the societal process of innovation in health the very nature and the characteristics of innovation change, a process that has been described as "the innovation of innovation." This leads further to the concepts of "open innovation" and "fluid innovation," which are discussed further below in relation to policy innovations for health [23].

In Switzerland a recent survey asked a group of health experts to identify the key technological and social drivers of innovation in health [24]. In the first category the experts established a ranking in the following order: (1) developments in biotechnology and genetics, (2) medical technology, (3) informatics and soft ware, (4) organic chemistry, (5) telecommunications and (6) nano technology. In the second category they ranked (1) demography, (2) individual responsibility, (3) nutrition, (4) education, and (5) income distribution. Most interesting though – and symptomatic for the speed of social change – is that the experts ranked the social driving forces as more important and forceful than the technological ones. Additionally they did not assign a high impact value to political driving forces – which reflects the assumption of the experts, that not much innovation is to be expected from traditional types of health policy.

The sociology of innovation argues that innovation itself has become a *Leitmotif* of 21st century society; this development is called "ubiquitous innovating" [25]. Indeed if one refers to some of the key documents – for example, of the European Union or of the OECD – a strategy for innovation is considered essential in order to compete in a global environment [3, 26]. It is interesting – with a view to liquid modernity – how similar the discussion of a new conceptualization of innovation is to the discussion on a new understanding of health. Health in turn is increasingly seen as one of the cornerstones for competitiveness and innovation. And like innovation it is increasingly seen to be in need of a policy approach that is more concerned with sustainability and long-term effects.

Box 3
Health sustainability challenges of 21st century societies

The key health sustainability challenges of 21st century societies are:

1. The demographic and financial pressure brought to bear on health and
    social systems through the ageing of societies – societies need to support
    an increase in healthy life expectancy and an independent life, despite
    disability and chronic disease; otherwise, we might witness a breakdown
    of support systems and social solidarities.
2. In view of new epidemiological developments – for example, the increase
    of overweight and obesity, early onset of diabetes, and an increase in
    mental health problems – the generation of children born at the turn of the
    21st century could be the first to have a lower health and life expectancy
    than their parents. Increased investment in the health of the next genera-
    tion is critical.
3. Health systems organization and financing is not sustainable without
    major reorientation away from acute care toward increased prevention,
    management of chronic disease, and community-based, integrated pri-
    mary health care.
4. With globalization we are witnessing the rapid spread and emergence
    of new infectious diseases – such as SARS and HIV AIDS – and the
    re-emergence of others, such as tuberculosis, there is increasing fear of
    a global influenza pandemic – increased preparedness is critical at all
    levels of health governance.
5. As 21st century societies are restructuring they are presently witnessing
    increasing health inequalities – addressing these widening gaps will be a
    key challenge for trust in modern democracies.
6. We are only just beginning to understand the health impacts of global
    warming and climate change – we must be more conscious of the
    interdependence of health sustainability and environmental sustainability
    [27].

Reconsidering the Territory of Health

While the territory of the medical system can be relatively clearly circumscribed
and framed in terms of delivery and utilization of health care services, the territory of health becomes ever less tangible and increasingly virtual. Disease has
boundaries; health does not. The new health challenges make this blatantly obvious.
Within government the stakeholders in the response to obesity are not only the health
ministry, but, for example, the ministries of transport, education, agriculture, trade,

and consumer affairs. Outside of government the producers of unhealthy food and drink products are as much in focus as are the settings of everyday life where they are consumed (such as canteens), global marketing and advertising practices, the media messages, and the role model celebrities to name but a few. Smoking acts regulate not only who can buy tobacco products, where, and at what price but they define where it is permitted to smoke; in consequence, owners of bars and restaurants, retailers, and the management of airports and railway lines to name but a few, all need to be concerned with health in ways they were not before. Consumers and voters as well as a wide array of health action groups and patient organizations make their preferences heard.

This infinite nature of health has consequences for all four domains of the health system. It is specific to the health society that all four domains – *personal health, public health, medical health,* and *the health market* – not only continue to change and expand but – and this is critical – that the balance between the systems is shifting [28]. The health sector – consisting of the public health domain and the medical health domain – struggles to include more health, in the form of strengthening public health, health promotion, and prevention. Yet, this approach is falling short in many countries, in particular for lack of political support, except where the measures are clearly medical, such as expanding screening or strengthening predictive medicine. While the new paradigms in preventative medicine are gaining increasing acceptance, public health measures are considered unduly paternalistic and are seen to impinge on the individual freedom of choice. Structural measures addressing the determinants are also not politically popular, as they usually impinge on one or the other economic interest. There have been excellent policy documents such as the Wanless Report in England [29] that have proposed to embark on an organizational shift within the health sector toward public health, driven in particular by the fear generated by the relentless growth of the medical health domain. They argue that more money needs to be invested in prevention, health promotion, and public health; otherwise, our societies will not be able to afford the constant expansion of the medical health system. So far within the health sector very few policies, institutions, organizations, and funding streams have clearly differentiated between investing for *health* and the expenditures for providing medical care. Durand-Zalesky makes this point in great detail in the contribution to this book and she underlines how important the political innovation environment is for a public health agenda focused on determinants – in the case of policy innovation for health the different perceptions of the role of the state, the market and the individuals are critical.

Where an accounting for health – which is different from the proposed national health accounts – is attempted, countries rarely reach more than a 2.9% average of the overall "health" budget for prevention, health promotion, and public health, as OECD data tell us [30]. Politically the pressure is strong to subject every penny of this paltry amount to critical evidence reviews based on a medical mind-set, while to this day most health service organizations are still not accountable for their health outcomes and demonstrate a severe lack of transparency for patients and consumers. It is therefore arguable whether the expansion of a traditional public health approach – for example, with more funding – will be sufficient. A new

Nordic Initiative argues – as do the authors in this book – that fundamentally new perspectives are needed. They locate them at three levels: mind-set, partnerships, and platforms [22].

Open Innovation: Involving a Broader Range of Actors

Policy innovations *for* health need to move beyond the established functional boundaries of both the medical health domain and the public health domain. The innovation debate can help in conceptualizing the necessary change. Open innovation is a term initially developed for the private sector and championed the idea that companies cannot anymore rely on their own innovative capacity – they need to share and outsource [31]. The perception of open innovation now means to involve a broad range of partners in order to find innovative solutions, particularly in the form of innovation clusters. As used to be the case in business, the functional and hierarchical approach in the medical and the public health domains do not usually allow for this. There are therefore very few policy mechanisms that allow decision makers to consider both health determinants and health impacts in an integrated manner and to approach the new health challenges with joined up policy responses, initiatives, and interventions. Usually each policy (sub) domain works to its own logic and intentions without regard for the impact on other areas of society or its global impact. Some exceptions can be found in the area of environmental policies.

If – with health in mind – we are willing to see the glass as half full, we can identify a range of policy innovations emerging in health that could be summarized under the term *network governance*. Examples are described in more detail in the chapter by Warner in this book. In many countries a first step to engage a broad range of actors around common goals was the development of health targets[32], an approach that gained ground from the 1980s onward. In order to achieve the targets it became clear that policies in the health sector needed to be complemented by other sectors of government and that they in turn needed to be supported by policy commitments at different levels of government and in the private and nongovernmental sector. The Wanless report calls this the *fully engaged scenario* [31]. In consequence a new type of policy mix is emerging between governmental measures, global initiatives, local action, consumer pressure and demand, and mechanisms – such as self-regulation or corporate social responsibility approaches – put into place by companies and the private sector.

Who would have imagined even a decade ago a range of the policy innovations for health we have witnessed recently:

- that a country would base its health policy on the determinants of health as in Sweden?
- that a health minister would regulate the body mass index of fashion models as in Spain?
- that television advertising of fast foods to children would be severely restricted as in England?
- that a country could accept a total ban on smoking in public places – including restaurants and bars as in Ireland?

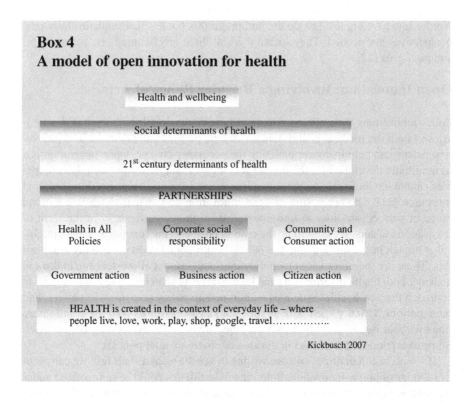

Box 4
A model of open innovation for health

Health and wellbeing

Social determinants of health

21st century determinants of health

PARTNERSHIPS

| Health in All Policies | Corporate social responsibility | Community and Consumer action |

| Government action | Business action | Citizen action |

HEALTH is created in the context of everyday life – where people live, love, work, play, shop, google, travel……………..

Kickbusch 2007

The health society not only means that health is present in every dimension of life, it also implies that risk is everywhere. As every place, setting, product or message in society can support or endanger health the potential stakeholders in any health policy decision expand exponentially; transport policies relate to the obesity epidemic, the beer tax influences young people's alcohol consumption and low literacy increases health inequalities.

Three types of policy innovations for health that qualify as open innovations are briefly outlined in the following: Health in All Policies, innovation clusters, and platforms.

"Health in All Policies"

A key policy innovation for health is the *Health in All Policies* approach put forward by the Finnish presidency of the European Union in 2006 [33] and first developed in the Ottawa Charter 1986 with the term "Healthy Public Policy" [17]. *Health in All Policies* is now also one of the four principles of the European Health Strategy of the EC [34]. I have described Health in All Policies as an innovative policy strategy that responds to the critical role that health plays in the economies and social lives of 21st century societies. It introduces better health (improved population health outcomes) and closing the health gap as shared goals across all parts of government and addresses complex health challenges through an integrated policy response across portfolios. By incorporating a concern with health impacts into the policy development process of all sectors and agencies, it allows government to address the key determinants of health in a more systematic manner, while taking into account the benefit of improved population health for the goals of other sectors [35]. Some countries have tried to reflect such an approach by creating a ministerial mechanism for the focus on health rather than disease; for example, Canada for a while had a minister for public health with cabinet rank, and England and Sweden both have junior ministers for *health*.

Innovation Clusters

Many partnerships are emerging beyond the health sector and its narrow policy conception. Increasingly we see a wide range of innovation clusters developing which create a new type of interface between many different actors following the open innovation model for companies but expanding it into public–private partnerships. One such example "Berlin's health care market" is described in this book in more detail by Henke and Martin. Another example is the "MyHeart" project – which brings 33 partners from 11 countries together to develop "intelligent textiles" in order to prevent heart disease [36] or the innovations in the area of functional foods. Of particular interest as a policy innovation for health is the proposal to establish "The Nordic region as a global health lab" [22]. It is proposed that the Nordic countries form an innovation cluster so that the Nordic region will become "a global market leader for prevention solutions." They further state that "the booming global market for health related products and services speaks in favor of joint initiatives, where knowledge and experiences produced within a research framework can be used to develop products and solutions attractive to the Nordic as well as the global market." They then go on to define the nine components that will give such an initiative a global competitive edge:

Box 5 The Nordic region as a global health lab

Nine components for success:

1. A social model supporting equal access to health for all
2. Prevention as a top Nordic policy priority
3. Access to valuable data
4. Strong civil society organizations
5. Strong conditions for collaboration
6. Innovative science environments
7. Strong industries
8. A competitive Nordic region
9. Demanding consumers provide a strong platform for user driven innovations

This initiative is a clear example of the attempt to build an innovation on a supportive policy environment in order to create social and economic value through health not only locally, but globally.

Platforms

Another move toward policy innovations for health based on open innovation approaches is the ever increasing number of platforms, coalitions, alliances, and networks built around health issues. A good example is the *European Platform on Diet, Physical Activity and Health* initiated in 2005 by the DG Sanco of the European Commission, which allows the commission to work with a wide range of players across the public, private, and nongovernmental sectors [37]. The stated intent is to create a platform for concrete actions designed to contain or reverse current trends, platform members must commit to action. As underlined in the White Paper on Strategy for Europe on Nutrition, Overweight and Obesity Related Health Issues, the Commission considers that the development of effective partnerships must be the cornerstone of Europe's response to tackling nutrition, overweight and obesity, and their related health problems. In such platforms the members agree to monitor and evaluate the performance of commitments in a transparent, participative and accountable way; the EU Platform, for example, works to a founding member's statement, has a monitoring framework and produces progress reports. The visibility and legitimacy conferred through such alliances is gaining increasing importance as a policy mechanism as are a myriad of public–private partnerships. Actors and issues gain prominence through media presentation and public debate as the health society is also a media-driven society. These platforms constitute a new political space for health and network governance, particularly for very controversial issues. The European Commission, for example, uses a multistakeholder platform to address alcohol issues through an "Alcohol and Health Forum," bringing together civil society and businesses pledging to take action to reduce alcohol-related harm in Europe [35].

The Democratization of Innovation: The Co-Production of Health

Innovation and knowledge are interdependent. Innovation can be defined as the process through which social and economic value is created through knowledge, an issue discussed in more detailed in the chapter by Sakellarides. This is done by different forms of knowledge creation, diffusion, transformation, and application. Both health and innovation are increasingly dependent on the inclusion of the user and challenged by the democratization of knowledge production. The sociology of innovation describes the innovation paradox, which postulates that in the knowledge society the role of the producer and the role of the consumer move ever closer together – health as well as innovation therefore need to be considered as coproduced goods [24]. In the area of technological innovation this is often described with terms like open source, open content, lead user, open innovation, collective invention, user innovation, and creative commons [38].

In health policy this participatory element has been neglected. On the one hand it is particularly difficult for the health care system to accept participation, because it has been defined by a very strong hierarchy between the professional physician, other health professionals, and the patient. Yet the management of chronic disease and the adherence to prevention regimes can only be achieved with full participation of the individual concerned. The overlap of unmet medical needs and unmet social needs can only be addressed jointly between patients, providers, and the social support system – patient input is a prerequisite to developing the kind of integrated disease-management models that most health systems still do not provide because they are out of step with the epidemiological and social development. The unmet medical and social need has led to the creation of a wide range of highly active patient organizations and self-help groups who act as the experts on "their" disease. The same applies to prevention and health promotion – the active participation of the individual, social groups, and communities is needed to engage in successful initiatives [39].

Sakellarides in his chapter highlights to interdependence of the knowledge society with innovation in the health society. Patients want information, participation, and choices – this is the result of the "European Patient of the Future" survey from 2003 [40]. Consumers want simplicity, convenience, speed, and a good price [41]. Increasingly the two expectations meet as health systems become increasingly market driven and as patients want more say and have higher expectations. New products and technologies can only develop their full potential if they meet processes and structures that allow them to do so. This implies new forms of information, communication, and integration processes. The Conference Board of Canada in its recent analysis [2] defines three dimensions of high performing health systems: people and culture, technologies, and structure and processes. This is also reflected in the more recent literature on innovation which speaks of a paradigm shift toward a "fluid identity of innovation" [42]. This means the "old" debates as to what constitutes a radical innovation and an incremental innovation is considered less and less relevant. This is often much more obvious in other, less regulated areas than the health sector.

A good example from information technology is the telephone: at what point in the long process from Graham Bell's machine to the tiny multifunctional mobile instruments we use today do we speak of radical or incremental innovation? When it turned wireless? When it could take photographs? When it became the iPhone? Whatever it will be in future? Similar questions arise in relation to medicines and medical technology which with the rise of chronic disease fulfill more than their primary medical function – they cannot cure any more so they will seek to reduce pain and the progress of disease, lengthen life, improve mobility, ensure independence, be easy to use, etc. The innovation process around medicines for HIV/AIDS is a typical case in point – every small improvement in the lives of AIDS patients counts and it continues to be driven not only by medical innovation but a very strong demand from influential user and advocacy groups.

Probably one of the most important process innovations that needs to be achieved lies in the transparency and accountability of health policy and health systems. Hernandez-Aguado in his chapter indicates how new types of monitoring could provide transparency and accountability for the impact that other sectors have on health. Sakellarides and his coauthors highlight the significance of patient-driven and patient-owned health information, also including the determinants of health. It is indeed worrying that in modern democracies, citizens – once they become patients – do not have access to data on the performance of the system that they enter or even to their own health data. This knowledge-based value creation will – as Sakellarides states – probably be the most relevant health policy innovation in the next decade. Health Consumer Powerhouse regularly publishes a ranking which indicates in which countries consumers and patients have the most rights and the most opportunities for participation [43]. A recent German survey showed that most citizens would like to see a ranking of physicians and would like to see their medical bills. [44]. If health is a coproduced good, then all those that participate in its production have a right to transparency of all elements of the process.

The issue of transparency also arises around propriety regulations. In the information technology field, there has been a move toward open access, open source, and open standards, and with the expansion of the Internet it has led to new forms of information access and sharing – the exciting mix of social and technological innovation, as reflected in platforms such as MySpace and Second Life. These demand-push innovations have in turn led to highly profitable companies. Due to the structure of the proprietary industry and government regulations, much of this innovation process remains closed. It is regularly challenged, in particular, by nongovernmental organization in relation to global health issues innovations – and more recently by the establishment of government assessment agencies. This conflict is not the subject of this book – yet it is worth referring to an interesting experiment at the World Economic Forum in 2006, which discussed how the break down of proprietary rights in the entertainment industry could be a signal for the pharmaceutical industry to reconsider its approaches with a new and proactive demand-push approach. In some cases this has succeeded at the global level where new forms of pricing, patent policies, and financing of pharmaceutical innovation for diseases of the developing world have been developed, and after much conflict a new cooperation between advocacy groups, the industry, governments, and modern philanthropy has emerged.

Outlook

For this book the key issue is that health is no longer a given; it is produced, maintained, and enhanced. The results of health research are rapidly transported through the media – a new cure, a new method of prevention, a new confirmation of old behaviors, all have high currency in the health society. What is considered healthy today might not be so tomorrow – new risks continuously emerge [45]. As a consequence heath literacy plays a critical role [46]. Risks are frequently not visible or seem intangible and they need to be well communicated, and above all understood and translated into action. As more and new health information becomes available this can become a difficult challenge for ordinary citizens in particular if they are not well educated or even functionally illiterate, as about 20% of all citizens in the OECD countries are. The expansion of health choices and the complexity of health systems demand an ever higher degree of sophistication and participation, and as a consequence there is a growing offer and demand not only for health information but for advice and knowledge brokering.

To be a passive and compliant patient who follows the physician's instructions is no longer sufficient – particularly when related to preventative issues. Indeed the emerging model is one of active and critical consumers, an ideal that only few members of the population can aspire to achieve. Already today – despite the universal access to health care – health inequalities abound even in the richest countries, and there is a clear danger that they will widen even further as the health society expands. The very presence of health in all areas of everyday life can also lead to a variety of reactions – either to attempts to reach an unrealistic body image or to conscious risk taking in opposition to an overpowering set of health messages and expectations. While the health society offers many opportunities of empowerment, it can also be prescriptive and exert social control through health [47]. Within a health society there has to be constant democratic dialog about the societal value we attach to health, a debate that has barely begun. Providing access to information on health and new health products and services including e-health is only a small part of the issues at stake as Sakellarides points out in his chapter. There is in general a big democratic deficit in relation to health and health policy, which needs to be addressed with urgency: the reorientation toward participation and user involvement will be one of the most important governance shifts in health.

What will innovation in health policy imply in the 21st century? If innovation means a *reorganization of how we approach health in 21st century societies,* I propose that the following five dynamic processes will be critical. Our societies will need to

- Develop a new understanding of health as an investment and productive force in society
- Develop separate governance mechanisms for health and for health care, with a strong focus on accountability for health gain
- Augment the concern for ethics and values with respect to health through a broad dialogue with citizens in order to increase democratic legitimacy and ensure solidarity
- Move beyond a narrow understanding of health outcomes in terms of only physical health measures to those that aim to include or even prioritize broader measures of wellbeing
- Engage in network governance, partnership and multi-stakeholder approaches in rder to achieve health goals.

The big 21st century health challenges call for more courageous and democratic policy approaches than applied so far. While our societies have now learned to recognize the urgency of the environmental challenge in terms of long-term sustainability, we are only just beginning to grasp the consequences that our way of life has in terms of health sustainability. An example of developing such a change in mindset are the 10 Health in All Policy principles developed in the South Australian Government in 2007 through a Health in All Polices process [35].

Box 6 Health in All Policies: the ten principles

A "Health in All Policies" approach reflects health as a shared goal of all of government. In particular, it

1. Recognizes the value of health for the well-being of all citizens and for the overall social and economic development of South Australia. Health is a human right, a vital resource for everyday life and a key factor of sustainability.
2. Recognizes that health is an outcome of a wide range of factors – such as changes to the natural and built environments or to social and work environments – many of which lie outside the activities of the health sector and require a shared responsibility and an integrated and sustained policy response across government.
3. Acknowledges that all government policies can have positive or negative impacts on the determinants of health and such impacts are reflected both in the health status of the South Australian population today and in the health prospects of future generations.
4. Recognizes that the impacts of health determinants are not equally distributed among population groups in South Australia and aims at closing the health gap, in particular for the Aboriginal peoples.
5. Recognizes that health is central to achieving the objectives of the South Australian Strategic Plan – it requires both the identification of potential health impacts and the recognition that good health can contribute to achieving South Australia Strategic Plan targets.
6. Acknowledges that efforts to improve the health of all South Australians will require sustainable mechanisms that support government agencies working collaboratively to develop integrated solutions to current and future policy challenges.
7. Acknowledges that many of the most pressing health problems of population health require long-term policy and budgetary commitment as well as innovative budgetary approaches.
8. Recognizes that indicators of success will be equally long term and that regular monitoring and intermediate measures of progress will need to be established and reported back to South Australian citizens.

9. Recognizes the need to regularly consult with citizens to link policy changes with wider social and cultural changes around health and well-being.
10. Recognizes the potential of partnerships for policy implementation between government at all levels, science and academia, business, professional organizations, and nongovernmental organisations to bring about sustained change.

An additional complexity is due to the fact that health in the 21st century is inherently global and many determinants of health are no longer in the control of nation states. Global and regional agreements of an economic and political nature can seriously endanger health – as experienced in rising alcohol rates in Finland and Sweden when they joined the European Union – or they can move the health agenda forward through transnational and global health agreements. The last 5 years have seen the acceptance by the WHO Member States of both the International Health Regulations and the Framework Convention on Tobacco Control. But other less binding approaches, such as the forceful move on a global strategy to combat chronic diseases, the policy by the European Union to consider the health impacts of all policies of the EU, the discussions on health at the Davos World Economic Forum, the new priority assigned to health in the OECD, and the product shift of many global companies, all illustrate the global driving force that health has become. Concerns arise around the global pharmaceutical market as much as over the global spread of sugary soft drinks, the global movement of health professionals as much as over the rapid global spread of viruses [48]. While the policy innovations for health required at the global level are not subject of this book, the authors are aware that this global nature of health is in itself one of the most significant driving forces of the reorganization of health in the 21st century.

Note by the author

Some parts of this chapter are based on a working paper for the Academic Advisory Group, which provided the guidance for the work on this publication. It was published as an editorial. (Kickbusch I. Innovation in health policy: responding to the health society. Gac San 2007;21:338–342).

Others draw on the opportunities available to me during my residency as the Adelaide Thinker in Residence in 2007. www.thinkers.sa.gov.au/ikickbusch.html

References

1. Gapper, J. OECD Observer Magazine Daily Summary. OECD Forum 2007 Innovation, Growth and Equity, Paris France 14–15. May 2007 www.oecd.org/document/35/0,3343,en_21571361_37578380_38597987_1_1_1_1,00.html accessed 15.03.2008.

2. Prada G., Santaguida P. (2007) *Exploring Technological Innovations in Health Systems*. Conference Board of Canada
3. OECD Health and Innovation Survey. www.oecd.org/document/10/0,3343,en_2825_495642_33790794_1_1_1_1,00.html accessed 15.03.2008.
4. Kickbusch, I. Health Governance: The Health Society. In: McQueen, D., Kickbusch I. et al. (2007) *Health and Modernity*. New York, Springer, 144–161.
5. Giddens, A. (1990) *The Consequences of Modernity*. Stanford, Stanford University Press.
6. Baumann, Z. (2005) *Liquid Life*. Cambridge, Polity Press.
7. McQueen, D., Kickbusch I. et al. (2007) *Health and Modernity*. New York, Springer.
8. Hesselbein F, Goldsmith M, Somerville I, (editors) (2001) *Leading for Innovation: & Organizing for Results*. Jossey Bass.
9. Marmot M., Wilkinson R. (2005) *Social Determinants of Health*. Oxford, Oxford University Press.
10. Health and Consumer Protection Directorate (2005) *The Contribution of Health to the Economy of the European Union*. Luxembourg
11. Foresight (2007) *Tackling Obesity – Future Choices Project Report*. www.foresight.gov.uk/Obesity/obesity_final/17.pdf accessed 20.03.2008.
12. National Institute of Public Health (2003) *Sweden's New Health Policy*. Stockholm
13. Public Health Agency of Canada: *Determinants of Health*. www.phac-aspc.gc.ca/ph-sp/phdd/determinants/index.html accessed 20.03.2008.
14. www.thewellbeingproject.org/wb/wellbeing_info.htm
15. World Health Organization (WHO) (1948) *Constitution*
16. The Ottawa Charter (1986) www.who.int/hpr/NPH/docs/ottawa_charter_hp.pdf
17. Whitelaw S, Baxendale A, Bryce C, MacHardy L, Young I and Witney M (2001) 'Settings' based health promotion: a review. Health Promotion International 16(4) 339–353.
18. Moulaert, F. and Sekia, F. (2003) Territorial innovation models: a critical survey. Regional Studies 37(3) 289–302.
19. www.worldvaluessurvey.org/
20. *Canadian Index of Wellbeing*. www.atkinsonfoundation.ca/ciw
21. The Nordic region as a global health lab. (2007) *NordForsk by Monday Morning*. www.nordforsk.org/pubinfo.cfm?pubid=67
22. Schumpeter S., Joseph A. (1964) Theorie der wirtschaftlichen Entwicklungen (6. Auflage, ursprünglich 1911). Berlin, Duncker und Humblot.
23. Braun-Thürmann, H. (2005) *Innovation*. Bielefeld, Transkript Verlag
24. Sigrist Sigrist, Stefan (2007) Wandel im Gesundheitsmarkt: strategische Ausrichtung der Pharma- und Biotechindustrie auf künftige Marktbedingungen und träventive Therapien. Dissertation, ETH Zürich
25. de.wikipedia.org/wiki/Innovation
26. EU Lisbon Strategy Europäische Union, (2000, 2005) Lissabon Strategie. ec.europa.eu/growthandjobs/index_de.htm accessed 12.02.2008.
27. Kickbusch I. (2008) *Healthy Societies*. Report Adelaide Thinker in Residence, Adelaide.
28. Kickbusch I. (2006) Die Gesundheitsgesellschaft. Gamburg Verlag, Gesundheitsförderung.
29. Wanless Report (2004) *Securing Good Health for the Whole Population*. HM Treasury. www.hm-treasury.gov.uk/consultations_and_legislation/wanless/consult_wanless04_final.cfm
30. Organisation for Economic Co-operation and Development, OECD Health Data 2006. *Statistics and Indicators for 30 Countries*. CD ROM and User's Guide, Paris 2006.
31. Chesbrough, H. W. (2003) *Open Innovation*. Boston, Harvard Business School Press.
32. Marinker M. (ed.) (2002) *Health Targets in Europe*. BMJ Books, London.
33. Kickbusch I., McCann W., Sherbon T. (2008) Adelaide revisited: from healthy public policy to Health in All Policies. In: *Health Promotion International*, 23(1), 1–4.
34. European Commission (2007) *Health Strategy White Paper*. ec.europa.eu/health/ph_overview/strategy/health_strategy_en.htm
35. Charter Establishing the European Alcohol Forum (2007) ec.europa.eu/health/ph_determinants/life_style/alcohol/documents/Alcohol_charter2007.pdf

36. MYHeart. *MyHeart Project. Fighting Cardio-Vascular Diseases by Prevention and Early Diagnosis*. www.hitech-projects.com/euprojects/myheart/ accessed 12.02.2008.
37. European Commission (2008) *EU Platform on Action on Diet, Physical Activity and Health*. ec.europa.eu/health/ph_determinants/life_style/nutrition/platform/platform_en.htm
38. Hippel E. von (2006) *Democratizing Innovation*. Cambridge MASS: MIT Press.
39. www.wkkf.org/Pubs/Health/TurningPoint/Pub3713.PDF
40. Coulter A., Magee H. (2003) *The European Patient of the Future. Picker Institute Europe*. www.isqua.org.au/isquaPages/Conferences/dallas/DallasAbstractsSlides/WebMaterial2003/PPT/Wednesday/C09/076_Coulter.pdf accessed 12.02.2008.
41. Schlögel M., Staib D., Feldmann L. *Black Box Kunde*, Gottlieb Duttweiler Institut, Rüschlikon (2004).
42. Khan M.R., Al Ansari M. (2005) Sustainable innovation as a corporate strategy. www.triz-journal.com/archives/2005/01/02.pdf
43. *Consumer Power House Health Consumer Powerhouse: Euro Health Consumer Index* (2007) www.healthpowerhouse.com/media/Rapport_EHCI_2007.pdf accessed 12.02.2008.
44. Böcken J., Braun B., Schnee M. (Hrsg.) Gesundheitsmonitor 2004. Die ambulante Versorgung aus Sicht von Bevölkerung und Ärzteschaft. Gütersloh: Verlag Bertelsmann Stiftung. www.bertelsmann-stiftung.de/cps/rde/xbcr/SID-0A000F14-7FC12C7F/bst/Inhalt_GeMo_2004.pdf accessed 12.02.2008.
45. Beck U. (1992) *Risk Society*. Cambridge, Polity Press.
46. Kickbusch I., Maag D. (2005) Health Literacy. Towards an active health citizenhip. In: Public Health in Österreich. Lengerich (Sprenger, M. (Hrsg)). Pabst Science Publishers, S.151–158.
47. Lupton D. (ed.) (1999) *Risk and Socio Cultural Theory, New Directions and Perspectives*. Cambridge, Cambridge University Press.
48. Bulletin of the World Health Organization. (2007) *Special Theme: Health and Foreign Policy*, 85(3) March.

Chapter 2
Intelligence for Health Governance: Innovation in the Monitoring of Health and Well-Being

Ildefonso Hernández-Aguado and Lucy Anne Parker

Abstract Good health governance requires appropriate health intelligence, and consequently, health information needs to be reshaped in order to foster health policy innovation. Several key aspects should pervade the new approaches to the management of health information: advocacy, monitoring broad health determinants, accountability, and transparency. Strong advocacy is needed if we wish to convince non-health sectors of the relevance of health in their policies. Successful advocacy is based on new and innovative ways of framing health information which contributes to moving health higher up the media, public, and policy agendas. The goal is to put across the effects that all societal sectors have on health and well-being. Advocacy in the terms mentioned is also required to transform public health from an underfunded pyramidal bureaucracy into a strengthened public health with higher-profile leadership. This represents a shift of approach from an individual-centred prevention linked to health services to a public health that makes healthy choices easier and is capable of promoting multifaceted policies from diverse sectors emerging through network governance.

We also propose the monitoring of the social determinants which have an established relationship with health. Health outcomes are usually the long-term effects of exposures that act during the whole life course. Consequently, in order to measure the effects of policies which take decades to manifest, we need to assess the evolution of health determinants addressed by these policies. In fact, responsibility for health is now so diffused at various levels and different sectors that it is very important to point out through appropriate information who is accountable for relevant health issues such as inequalities.

Health-related information should be produced and framed in a way that is suited to the relevant level of governance in order to target accountability and transparency. The aim is to identify what part of government (local, national, regional, or global) is accountable for any health-related issue. Recent innovations such as health impact assessment are the starting point for the development of policy-linked

I. Hernández-Aguado (✉)

Department of Public Health, Facultad de Medicina, Universidad Miguel Hernández, Campus de San Juan, 03550 Alicante, Spain
ihernandez@umh.es

I. Kickbusch (ed.), *Policy Innovation for Health*,
DOI 10.1007/978-0-387-79876-9_2, © Springer Science+Business Media, LLC 2009

indicators: "avoidable burden of disease by policies" or "health expectancy gained through policy." These indicators may be estimated at every governance level and are understandable to policy makers and to the public. Transparency and intelligibility of health information is a keystone for population engagement that brings about demands for political actions in health, and consequently should guide innovation in health monitoring.

Although, as far as possible, new policies must be evidence based, the absence of evidence is a stimulus to innovation. Future advances in the monitoring of health and well-being must combine research and implementation. The challenges are evaluation of complex social programs; proper surveillance of new policies with health effects; provision of good data on the economic and social effects of health investment; assurance of a high societal visibility of health issues; and engagement of all stakeholders in the call for accountability and transparency.

Introduction

Good health governance needs good information. However, are we not already overwhelmed with data, statistics, indicators, and all kinds of health information? Is not the insistence on measuring a result of classical and paralyzing epidemiology? Why devote efforts to the surveillance of health when emphasis on monitoring usually turns into an obstacle to policy implementation? There is no doubt that a myriad of initiatives on health information management exist at all levels of governance activity. However, there is a quality gap between health information on hand and the health information framed and provided to the stakeholders. This is our great challenge. In this chapter we describe the potential for innovation in health information management. We depict how appropriate health information could foster innovative health policies, particularly the initiatives linked to Health in All Policies (HiAP).

The process of setting population health targets sought to shift the focus of the health world from inputs to outcomes [1]. Nevertheless there has been a permanent tension between target setting for health based on simple etiological views and driven by behavioral epidemiology and target setting that takes up the complex political and social processes needed to tackle the root causes of ill health. In the words of Kickbusch:

> increasingly target setting became a technocratic/professional/managerial enterprise rather than a process to set in motion the acceptance of new political priorities for health policy, in order to define and ensure the new health territory. Indeed, recent experiences in England show that while targets at first seem to be an ideal approach to monitor accountability and performance at various levels of the health system, their "overuse" can become counterproductive and unmanageable as time is spent on reporting rather than on implementing policy [2].

Appropriate health information needs to be parallel to policy making instead of a hindrance. The new health governance acknowledges the fact that action is needed in and by sectors other than health and requires health information that contributes to this new approach.

We first outline some of the key factors that health information should satisfy for better health governance.

Health information should be framed in a way that supports advocacy for Health in All Policies by moving health higher up the media, public, and policy agendas. Durand-Zaleski, in her chapter, calls for policy-maker motivation in supporting the Health in All Policies approach by cutting across existing beliefs and bureaucratic territories. Therefore, the rationale and needs of sectors other than health should be considered when designing information systems and indicators.

The policies of the new health governance should address social determinants of health and consider the powerful long-term health effects of policies dealing with specific risk in critical life course paths such as child development and transition of young adults to the workforce. Information is required in order to indicate what part of government or society is accountable for inequalities and other social determinants of health.

The need for health accountability is expanding parallel to the expansion of the territory of health. Many sectors across society are accountable for health both in positive and negative terms. Health and well-being need new reporting formats which emphasize transparency and use opportune channels of information. Health-related information should reach a wide variety of stakeholders, decision makers from any sector, the public at large, etc. Citizen feedback and participation is a key component of health accountability and contributes to a central dimension of policy which is democracy. Marinker, when considering the values that underpin policy making, wrote of democracy that:

> In order to engender confidence in health policies, all stakeholders, and especially citizens and patients, need to be actively engaged. Access to health information and health literacy are crucial to such engagement. Health policies succeed in relation to the sense of solidarity and shared values that they foster [3].

The challenge is not so much transparency in the functioning of health services [4], but rather health information that contributes to a better awareness of the citizens of the determinants of their health and of the policies that affect these determinants. Health literacy plays a relevant role in policy innovation and is thoroughly considered elsewhere in this book.

Many actors could be involved in the new health governance. Any group or institution can lead initiatives for better health. This participatory policy process requires collaboration among a wide array of stakeholders. As Warner describes in his chapter, networks are more efficient in situations where the problems are complex and organizational effort fragmented. Flexible network-based mechanisms need health information that is suited to every policy level, that is linked to specific policies, and that monitors effects across sectors.

The chapter on health as an economic driver reports how evidence is accumulating on the relationship between health and wealth. However, there is still a lack of precise information that clearly illustrates the link between policies in non-health sectors that increase health level and which, as a consequence of this increase, contributes to other attainments such as productivity, efficiency, and so on.

In the second part of this chapter we review the different developments in health information so far implemented in developed countries. Starting from some innovative developments that relate health outcomes with risk factors and with policies, we propose in the third part a health information management which offers transparency and accountability, that encourages participation, and that is attractive to the decision makers in non-health sectors. Finally we consider the outlook for the future and point out the need for a good mix of research and implementation in order to make advances in the monitoring of health and well-being.

Part I: Health Information for Governance Innovation

From Ottawa Charter to Health in All Policies

The effect that policies from diverse sectors have on health has long since been acknowledged. Regulations concerning environment, housing or transport, among other areas, are part of health protection. Moreover, advocating for health through influence on education, nutrition, or social affairs has been at the core of health promotion, particularly the healthy cities movement [5]. However, the dominance in the health policy field of the health care sector, together with the scant power of public health specialists and researchers to influence policies, hinders the full development of new health policy approaches. On the other hand, many public health specialists remain aloof from the values shared by those tackling upstream determinants of health and are prone to follow the classic risk factor approach of epidemiology leading to interventions centred on the individual and mainly based on the conventional health education.

The Ottawa Charter in 1986 conceptualized health as "a resource for living," proposed a shift of focus from disease prevention to "capacity building for health," and established as one key action "building healthy public policy" [6]. With this backup, health promotion has unrelentingly accumulated experience over more than 20 years seeking to move away a focus on individual behaviors to the population approach suggested by Geoffrey Rose [7].

The ideas that arose from the initial steps of health promotion initiatives became popular in certain professional, academic, and institutional circles, but in spite of their solid bases, they remained alien to the main stream of the health sector. Influencing non-health sectors appeared beyond reach. However, health promotion has been characterized by its determination and tenacity and new and diverse strategies have been frequently tested in order to overcome the barriers to change and to accomplish public health aspirations through multifaceted policies. A healthy public policy had been characterized by its explicit concern for health and equity in all areas of policy and by accountability for health impact. The main aim was to create supportive environments to enable people to lead healthy lives [8].

Parallel to the multiple health promotion initiatives the population approach to health has been reinforced by the increased attention from the epidemiological world to the root determinants of health. In the last decade there has been an increase in epidemiological research on social determinants of health. Social epidemiology has moved the focus from the individual causes of disease to the population determinants [9–15]. Broad approaches to understanding the upstream causes of ill health have highlighted the interrelation between health and other spheres of society. Consequently, these initiatives have lead to the recognition that interventions addressing upstream roots of health problems lie outside the health domain.

The parallel and positive trajectories of health promotion and population health research have contributed to the promotion of healthy public policies. Gradually the approach of placing health criteria on the agendas of policy makers who have not previously considered health as a relevant issue is climbing the ladder of institutional and public recognition. This vision of health policy has received a major boost at the European level with the initiative "Health in All Policies" (HiAP) of the Finnish presidency [16]. One key argument for the HiAP proposal is that health is a requirement for production, the main aim of European policies being the growth, employment, and innovation. The need for a new policy model is even clearer at the global level where it has been stated that the crisis in global health is not a crisis of disease but a crisis of governance [17]. HiAP gives health a key role in the 21st century societies by including health gains and a reduction in health gaps as shared goals of all government departments. With this approach, health determinants become a concern of public policies in all sectors that can address them in a more systematic way.

The endorsement at high political level of the principles that are at the heart of the population health approaches should be viewed as a window of opportunity to support change and policy innovation. Whether or not this innovative policy approach will succeed, and to what degree, will depend on a great array of combined initiatives among which the management of health information could be relevant.

Initiatives on Health Information Management

Monitoring health and health information management is linked to the foundation of public health and is the mainstay of any public health activity. As has been noted, *"a clear, permanently updated, picture of what is in fact happening out there is essential"* [18]; good health governance requires appropriate health intelligence and this recognition could partially explain the recent upsurge of interest in health information and health statistics. At the global level, the work of the WHO through the World Health Organisation Statistical Information System (WHOSIS) is of great value. On the other hand, the worldwide increase in health and other development initiatives have prompted the need for appropriate health information systems able to guide an effective allocation of resources. Public and private agencies involved in international funding require health information to sustain political and financial support for their programs. This is particularly relevant in developing countries and is well illustrated by the problems found in monitoring the Millennium Development Goals (MDGs). The issue has been extensively addressed by a series in The Lancet on Health Statistics [19–22].

At the regional level (multinational) there are also several initiatives from international institutions concerned with health information. In developed countries the Organisation for Economic Co-operation and Development (OECD) carries out valuable work in the field of health monitoring, analyzing different proposal of indicators, and testing their relation with social and economic measurements [23]. We should also highlight the European Community Health Indicators (ECHI) projects under the European Health Monitoring Programme that have developed a comprehensive list of indicators in order to accomplish three general objectives: to monitor trends throughout the EU, to evaluate EU policies, and to enable international comparisons [24]. The European Commission also has its own office of statistics, Eurostat, that provides regular data and indicators for the monitoring of health and well-being [25].

Among the national initiatives we can distinguish among several proposals with different underlying visions of public health. For instance, worth mentioning are the proposal of indicators for monitoring the new Swedish public health policy [26] and the proposition by the Centres for Disease Control and Prevention (CDC) in the USA [27].

Space for Innovation in Health Information

With this myriad of initiatives, efforts and projects related to the monitoring of health and well-being, one can hardly discern any space for innovation. Moreover, beyond the above-mentioned initiatives, many countries have regular reports on population health and health determinants at different administrative levels as well as other traditional and firmly established public health surveillance systems. Before reaching hasty conclusions about the potential for innovation, it is worth remembering that, in spite of the overwhelming quantity of health data and information, critical features are lacking. These include the related features of accountability and transparency that are central to good governance (Box 1).

Box 1. Accountability and transparency

Health information and accountability

Acknowledgment and responsibility for actions, decisions, or policies is possible if the resulting consequences can be reported and explained. Policy accountability is more likely if a time connection between the policies and their health effects can be established.

Available health monitoring systems and health reports do not reveal who or what policies are responsible for our current levels of healthy life expectancy or self-perceived health. In fact most health outcomes measured have many diverse determinants that influence health throughout the life course of populations and which are modified mainly by non-health policies.

Most government areas should be accountable for the present and future levels of population health but most of the decision makers in these areas are not aware of this responsibility. There is a need to produce and frame health information that reveals the health benefits (or detriments) that can be attributed to a specific policy change. This will require a wise use of data and evidence to provide measurable outcomes that are modifiable by policies and on that in turn may predict health outcomes.

Health information and transparency

Transparency is a key element of accountability and means that implementation of policies and activities is carried out in a manner that can be easily observed and understood by the relevant stakeholders and particularly the public. While accountability refers to the consequences of actions or decisions, transparency enables the public not only to assess the outcomes of decisions but also to observe and participate during or before the decision-making process.

Transparency implies appropriate response to requests for information and good quality of reporting to the public and stakeholders. The health care sector is now emphasizing transparency by ensuring that the public have access to information on the quality of care they receive from providers. However, this is not at all a universally implemented and accepted policy.

Transparency in policy process could be enhanced if health information management generated clear reporting of the predictive health outcomes derived from diverse policy options that are easily understandable to policy makers and to the public at large.

For example, it is theoretically acknowledged that health systems should be governed and evaluated by the production of health and reduction of disease; however, the public in many countries do not usually have access to performance indicators of hospitals and other health care services that measure health outcomes. Furthermore, many health policies have long-term consequences and it is difficult to establish a clear connection between their implementation and their effects. Understandably, the health effects of non-health policies are even less frequently assessed and evaluation of the effects of health investments in productivity terms or other societal attainments is rarely carried out. On the other hand, health and well-being have become a central aspect of everyday life but insufficient attention is paid to the measurement process by governments and other stakeholders. To illustrate this point, consider the high volume of daily and monthly economic data, statistics, and information that flood the media and, on the other hand, the unavailability of a clear and regularly updated picture of the level of satisfaction and well-being of the population.

The lack of accountability and transparency in the management of health information hampers good health governance. These principles should guide any proposal for innovation. Box 2 shows some of the potential contributions of health information management to facilitate the implementation of innovative health policies. Some of the points displayed are considered in other chapters of this book. In this chapter, we will mainly focus on points 1 and 3 to 6.

Box 2. Health information bases for policy innovation

1. Health information framed in a way that recognizes the value of health for the well-being of all citizens and for the attainment of many societal objectives
2. Monitoring of the distribution of health determinants across of the different social sectors of society
3. Design of attractive means to show the impact on health of all government policies including inaction
4. Development of health and well-being indicators that induce accountability and transparency, both for the health sector and the non-health sector
5. Identification of indicators of progress linked to the intermediate effects of policies on all sectors that have an effect on health
6. Assessment of the density of policies that are guided under the principles of Health in All Policies
7. Monitoring of citizens' vision of health and well-being issues
8. Creation of mediating structures in order to improve knowledge transfer
9. Contribution to health literacy and participation of the population

Advocacy Through Innovative Health Information Framing and New Indicators

One key aspect of future health information management is its potential contribution to an increase in the relevance of health in all public policy. Establishing health as a public good and placing Health in All Policies requires particular attention to the process of moving health higher up the agenda and taking advantage of windows of opportunity to change policy. This is a challenge relevant to every decision level and any success fuels the development at the other levels. For example, if the present European health strategy [28] succeeds in achieving greater HiAP cooperation and as a result HiAP becomes a common practice in some European countries, the achievement will inspire and stimulate this new governance in other countries and encourage other administrative levels to follow. At the same time the success could help in strengthening the European voice in global health. On the other hand, demonstrations of policy achievements at local level reinforce national and international strategies.

Advocacy is specifically one of the key applications of health indicators and has, as any other public health action, the ultimate goal of improving population health. While advocacy is an understandable consequence of obvious health problems revealed by health information systems or health indicators, too often health information is swallowed up in the stream of competing information space. Hence, in order to place health in the media, public, and policy agendas, new and innovative ways of framing health information, are needed, particularly if we wish to convince non-health sectors of the relevance of health in their policies. Advocacy of innovative health policies could be supported if we report opportune information that links any policy with its health effects and also if we can show the effects of health investments in any other societal domains (Box 3).

Box 3. Advocacy

Advocacy and health information

Advocacy is the act of taking a position on an issue, and initiating actions in a deliberate attempt to influence private and public policy choices [29]. Success in developing healthy public policies requires, among other factors, efforts in public health policy.

Development of Health in All Policies will depend on the players involved: policy makers, policy influencers, the public and the media. Key policy influencers are the public health practitioners, their associations, and other organizations with common objectives (for example, reduction of poverty, contamination control, safe neighborhoods, and so on).

Public health advocacy works through the media and other channels in order to influence policy makers and the public. The understanding and attitudes of the public towards the health question affect the adoption of the policy.

Health information can be used by relevant interest groups to encourage and influence the policy change. Furthermore, proper advocacy through good information framing must be capable of pointing out not only the health effects of any desired non-health policy but also the effects that the health gains have on other social and economic domains.

The Value of Well-Being for the Attainment of Many Societal Objectives

The strategy of placing Health in All Policies may be hindered by the main goals of government policy. For example, the Lisbon Strategy of the European Union underlines competitiveness as one of its fundamental goals. This emphasis may mean that health is far from being a priority of other policies, but that health policy is subordinated to economical and industrial policies. The key challenge is to highlight the synergies that make health a priority in all policies, in other words, ensure that questions related to health are seen as assets in the achievement of underlining economic targets. Moreover, making health an objective should be seen as socially and politically advantages. Therefore, we require information that shows clearly the links between health and well-being, between both of these and varying social and economical goals.

Some knowledge is already available which relates, for example, improvements in occupational health to business productivity and competitiveness targets. Our task now is to gather disperse data and present it in ways that contribute to optimize communication and advocacy. The general public must be made aware of the importance of health and well-being in the achievement of societal objectives. Health literacy in a broad sense (that is, awareness of what makes a population healthy and how good health impacts on societal attainments) could play a significant role in shaping policies. Efforts to increase health literacy as those described by Sakellarides in his chapter should embrace the spirit of HiAP and thereby enhance the engagement of the population in policy innovation.

An opportunity to measure and communicate well-being is that the economic sectors are interested in showing that policy making goes beyond economics, seeking to avoid trade-offs between economic and social policies and instead to encourage them to reinforce each other. In fact, few institutions wish to be seen as overemphasizing only economic goals. Measuring material living standards in terms of gross domestic product is not enough and other factors should be taken into account. Therefore, well-being and happiness are now becoming an important component of policy evaluation, at least rhetorically. This conclusion also emerges after reviewing a statistical paper from the OECD [30] and the presentations at the international conference in Rome on measuring happiness [31–33]. In this context, indicators become a central issue, and different approaches are being considered. Gross domestic product per family, composite indicators, happiness, and opportunities are among the latest proposals. Some of this work could be relevant for our purpose of finding indicators that on one hand are linked to health and sensitive to non-health policies, and on the other hand may show the effects of investment on health.

Measuring Outcomes That Are Relevant to Non-health Policies

Most of the indicators proposed for public health monitoring include outcomes related to health status. There is no doubt that mortality, morbidity, generic health status (perceived health, quality of life, etc.), and composite measures of health status (disability-free life expectancy, other life expectancies, etc.) should be at the core of any set of public health indicators as their improvement is the major endeavour of public health policies. Overall health status is the result of the mixed effects of all health determinants which have influenced health during the life course and – with some exceptions – it is not easy to establish the link between any single policy and health status, particularly in the case of non-health policies. Although some individual health indicators are sensitive to the effect of specific policies, this fact occurs unevenly according to type of policy.

It is worth remembering here the different concepts of public health that shape the types and targets of public health policies. Visions of public health range from an approach based on individual preventive medicine (including screening, immunization and medial counselling) to an approach derived from the principles of health promotion mentioned above, which constructs policies from the question: What makes people healthy? Individual-focused public health uses the so-called risk factor epidemiology and emphasizes change of behaviors. Population-focused public health stresses healthy public policy which is the basis of HiAP.

Broadening the scope of outcomes to be monitored is crucial if we wish to place health in other policies. Educational, agricultural, trade, social affairs, or occupational policies have primarily non-health outcomes but are frequently related to well-being and health. The challenge is to identify measurable targets of non-health policies that are closer to health and are sensitive to these policies.

Some health policies, those originating in health bureaucracies with health as their explicit and main objective, can be evaluated through their effect on specific health outcomes included in the usual collection of public health indicators. This is not the case for non-health policies, those aimed mainly at non-health objectives and whose effect in health operates indirectly through the general determinants of health. With some exceptions, the effect on health of non-health policies is not disease specific and consequently is hardly sensitive to monitoring by individual health indicators.

There is a paradox: while population health level is attributable mainly to socioeconomic and political context influenced by governance, macroeconomic policies, public policies – largely non-health policies, and culture and social values [34], we are apparently unable to monitor in the short term the effect on health of policies directed at these determinants. On the other hand, the usual broad-spectrum health indicators are more appropriate in measuring the general effects of the above-mentioned determinants and their related policies in the long term than in measuring the results of health policies. The evaluation of the overall health policy is attained by estimating the mortality considered amenable to health care before a specified age limit (e.g., 75) as has been recently reported for industrialized countries comparing present with earlier estimates [35].

Accountability: Can Single Indicators Make Policies More Accountable?

Focusing on some specific health policies, their effect can be monitored, as mentioned above, through single health indicators (either disease-specific mortality or special indicators). This is the case of cervical cancer incidence or mortality and avoidable hospital mortality. Cervical cancer screening can be monitored through its effect on cervical cancer incidence and mortality, while programs to reduce adverse events in hospital care can be evaluated by changes in avoidable hospital mortality. Therefore, cervical screening policies and quality of hospital care policies as well as other specific health policies can be assessed by adequate indicators that show their effects in terms of health outcomes. Nonetheless, we should not ignore the fact that even very specific health indicators are always sensitive to a series of factors and consequently any changes in the value of the indicator are due to changes produced by alterations in one or more of these involved factors.

Cervical cancer screening is a well-defined health intervention but interacts with socioeconomic factors and other policies that modify its effects. Many opportunistic cervical screening programs did not show any modification in cervical cancer mortality trends, and this was explained by the fact that those women frequently screened were those with the highest socioeconomic level and thus with the lowest risk. Only when screening programs are designed to have wide coverage is a downward trend in cervical cancer mortality observed [36]. Likewise, policies to improve quality of health care in hospitals are modified by the socioeconomic context that could affect the result of the interventions. Hence, many health outcomes apparently linked to well-defined health interventions take in the effects of other health determinants frequently shaped by non-health policies. However, we can barely use these selected indicators of health status, such as disease-specific or problem-specific mortality or incidence, to monitor non-health policies because the attributable proportion of disease to these policies is time and place dependent and commonly unknown.

There are some single health indicators that can be used to monitor the effect on non-health policies. Transport policies and environmental policies can have short-term effects on disease-specific mortality or morbidity. Nevertheless, we hold that this is not the rule: health outcomes reflect the results of many factors throughout a life course. They provide outcomes in the long term but are not explanatory of the etiologic process involved from the upstream level to the individual level. Their use in assessing non-health policies is very limited.

In summary, clearing a path for HiAP entails particular attention to information management. There is already a wide recognition of the relevance of health information at all governance levels. Consequently there is now a variety of initiatives that supply the public health community with numerous statistics and indicators that allow proper health monitoring. However, there is space for innovation mainly in how the health information is framed and provided to the relevant stakeholders. Many non-health policies have health effects through the modification of the social determinants of health and reduction of inequalities. The relevant results for the stakeholders of non-health policies are not primarily health outcomes, but rather the impact on the determinants mentioned. In order to use health information in advocacy of HiAP, new indicators and new ways of framing health information that clearly link non-health policies with intermediate outcomes and health are required. Health information innovation demands attention to the basic principles of accountability and transparency. In the second part of the chapter and considering these premises, we revise the state of the art in health information in order to build our proposals described in the third part.

Part II: Health Information Today: Current Strategies and Proposals for Health Indicators

Conceptual Framework

The use of health indicators in advocating for public health policies requires that the indicators have certain features. If by advocating we mean raising health up the political agenda and supporting the presence of Health in All Policies, the indicators chosen should measure those outcomes and determinants of health that are relevant to the conceptual framework shared by those that defend this vision of public health. In fact any proposal of indicators to monitor health reveals the vision of public health held by the authors. It has been acknowledged that while values are present in the preamble of almost every national health policy, they are less visible in the core text of these policies, describing action, resources, implementation, evaluation, and so on [37]. The central values can be involved in the setting of health targets [1] and as such the indicators chosen to monitor the health of the population should reflect them, allowing for the evaluation of progress. Although there may be a broad consensus on what is important, this does not always translate into practice and the proposals for indicators may reflect a limited consideration of these values. Indicators on health determinants might be completely absent, while sometimes there is only a narrow selection focusing on determinants of health that are restricted to the individual behaviors, and in some propositions there is a diverse range in both qualitative and quantitative terms, of the determinants being considered.

When reviewing the proposals of health indicators in developed countries, one can notice the degree of recognition by the authors of the contribution to health of social aspects, environment, and individuals.

Health Information at Regional Level

The case of the OECD is relevant as this institution is carrying out long-term research into population indicators exploring the relationship between economic and well-being measures [23]. The 2005 OECD report on health arranges indicators into five categories which, besides health status and health systems, include nonmedical determinants of health and demographic and economic context. It is noticeable that the nonmedical determinants section lists classical indicators of lifestyle behaviors such as tobacco and alcohol consumption or body weight while measurement of upstream determinants is omitted. On the other hand, the OCDE report on social indicators [38] does present indicators reflecting self-sufficiency, equity, and social cohesion involving financial, employment, social spending, and well-being measures (Table 1).

The European Union Public Health Programme has as a key objective to provide comparable information on the health of European citizens by developing

Table 1 Social indicators. Organisation for Economic
Co-operation and Development (OECD)

Self-sufficiency
Total employment rates.
People in jobless households.
Average years of schooling.
Mean student performance.

Equity
Income inequality.
Relative poverty rate.
Child poverty.
Gender wage gap.

Health
Healthy life expectancy at birth.
Life expectancy at birth (total).
Infant mortality.
Potential number of years lost.

Social cohesion
Volunteering.
Victimization rate.
Convicted adults.
Suicide rates.

health indicators and collecting data. According to their goals the information to be collected should cover the health-related behavior of the population (e.g., data on lifestyles and other health determinants), diseases (e.g., incidence and ways to monitor chronic, major and rare diseases), and health systems (e.g., data on access to care, on the quality of care provided, on human resources, and on the financial viability of healthcare systems). An essential feature of the European Union objectives is that the data collection should be based on comparable health indicators applicable to the whole of Europe, and on agreed definitions and methods of collection and use. Taking as a starting point the earlier work by international organizations such as WHO-Euro (Health for All database) and OECD, and working in close cooperation with them, several projects have been implemented to develop a set of common European health indicators. Among them the most exhaustive initiative is the previously mentioned European Community Health Indicators (ECHI) Project [24]. This project has drawn up two lists of indicators (short and long). Work on these indicators and the data collection is carried out by coordinated Working Parties, in cooperation with Eurostat and the Community Statistical Programme. The final objective of the European Union is to develop a European Union System of Health Information and Knowledge, which is fully accessible to European experts and the general public. For those who are engaged in highlighting broad determinants of health, it is critical the inclusion in this framework of indicators that take into account such upstream causes of ill health.

The final report of the European Community Health Indicators (ECHI) project (short list) proposes 82 indicators. Compared to the above-mentioned OECD health indicators, this proposal widens the scope of population health determinants by

Table 2 Main categories for the European Community Health Indicators set [24]

1 Demographic and socio-economic situation
1.1 Population
1.2 Socio-economic factors
2 Health status
2.1 Mortality
2.2 Morbidity, disease-specific
2.3 Generic health status
2.4 Composite health status measures
3 Determinants of health
3.1 Personal and biological factors
3.2 Health behaviours
3.3 Living and working conditions
4 Health systems
4.1 Prevention, health protection, and health promotion
4.2 Health care resources
4.3 Health care utilisation
4.4 Health expenditures and financing
4.5 Health care quality/performance

including socioeconomic factors and living and working conditions (Table 2). However, it is remarkable that the final proposal (long or short) gives so little importance to broad health determinants in comparison to indicators of health service activities or health outcomes.

Another European Project (European Union Health Promotion Indicator Development (EUHPID)) recognized the substantial lack of indicators on health promotion activities in the ECHI proposal. In line with their different conceptual model, they adapted the section on health systems, splitting it as follows: (1) Health interventions: health services (2) Health interventions: health promotion [39]. This is shown in Table 3, together with the a selection of indicators illustrating the choice of indicators on health determinants included in the ECHI short list.

In addition to this slight modification, the authors of EUHPID Project recognize that the ECHI list focuses largely on pathogenic and individual-level health development and on health care systems. They point out that this focus is paradoxical given the estimates that only 20% of life expectancy gain during the 20th century (reported for the United States) is due to improvements in health services, while the remaining 80% is due to changes in lifestyles and particularly to changes in the socioecological environment. For the future, they propose the development of complementary indicators emphasizing salutogenic health development in everyday life. However, they are more centred on individual outcomes (health capacities, sense of community, social capital, health literacy, and sense of coherence) than in identifying upstream determinants and health-related outcomes of non-health policies. In our view, the proposal from EUHPID highlights the need to monitor the result of actions implemented from the public health field although applied in diverse domains such as schools and workplaces, and their effects. The proposal does not consider

Table 3 Selected indicators extracted from the ECHI shortlist, divided by two grades of availability of data

Indicator class	Regularly available, reasonably comparable	Partly available, sizeable comparability problems
Demographic and socio-economic factors	• Population by gender/age • Birth rate • Mother's age distribution (incl. teenage pregnancies) • Fertility rate • Population projections • Population by education • Population by occupation	
Health determinants	• Regular smokers • Total alcohol consumption • Intake of fruit • Intake of vegetables • PM10 exposure	• Body mass index • Blood pressure • Pregnant women smoking • Hazardous alcohol consumption • Use of illicit drugs • Physical activity • Breastfeeding • Social support • Work-related health risks
Health interventions: health promotion	Policies against ETS exposure	• Policies on healthy nutrition • Policies/practices on lifestyles etc. • Integrated programmes in settings

explicitly the monitoring of the health effects of policies implemented outside the health sector and their results.

Health Information at National Level

The leading health indicators of the Healthy People 2010 initiative (Table 4) launched by the U.S. Department of Health and Human Services are mostly centred on individual behaviors and health status [27]. Although Healthy People 2010 encompasses 467 objectives in 28 focus areas and some objectives cover the effects of physical and social environments and the policies and interventions used to promote health, most objectives focus on specific health interventions that are individually oriented and designed to reduce or eliminate illness, disability, and premature death. Nonetheless, it is worth mentioning that the whole initiative takes in some of the recent developments in population health and social epidemiology.

As an example of a public health model that stresses the relevance of non-health data, the proposal of the New Swedish Public Health Policy stands out. The new

Table 4 Leading health indicators selected for Healthy People 2010 (U.S. Department of Health and Human Services) [27]

The Leading Health Indicators
• Physical activity
• Overweight and obesity
• Tobacco use
• Substance abuse
• Responsible sexual behaviour
• Mental health
• Injury and violence
• Environmental quality
• Immunization
• Access to health care

model seeks to monitor health determinants instead of health outcomes or health care indicators in an effort to provide more accessible information for political decisions. A committee including all parliamentary parties, a large number of research experts and other important interest groups produced a set of 11 general objectives (Table 5) with the intention of drawing up a public health policy report every 4 years and presenting developments in these key areas [40].

The first six objectives cover broader structural determinants reflecting the conditions in specific areas of society. The relevance of policy from non-health sectors is apparent. The last five objectives reflect lifestyle determinants, pertinent once again to the individual although in this case, in considering suitable indicators, the substantial role played by social environment is taken into account. In November 2004, 38 main indicators were adopted [26].

An important consideration is the acknowledgment of the need to stratify all indicators by sex, age, type of family, different administrative level, socioeconomic group, and ethnicity. This facilitates the monitoring of the primary value of promoting equity. To assess objective 1, "participation and influence in society," Swedish Public Health Policy proposes as indicators: the turnout in municipal elections, an index of gender equality, and the percentage of the population actively

Table 5 Eleven general objectives for the Swedish Public Health Policy [40]

1. Participation and influence in society
2. Economic and Social Security
3. Secure and favourable conditions during childhood and adolescence
4. Healthier working life
5. Healthy and safe environments and products
6. Health and medical care that more actively promotes good health
7. Effective prevention against communicable diseases
8. Safe sexuality and good reproductive health
9. Increased physical activity
10. Good eating habits and safe food
11. Reduced use of tobacco and alcohol, a society free from illicit drugs and doping, and a reduction in the harmful effects of excessive gambling.

employed. The key decision makers related to these indicators work outside the health service.

Under objective 3, "secure and favourable conditions during childhood and adolescence," they consider, among other things, the level of education of nursery employees. This shows a level of consideration far beyond the health state of children in preschool but acknowledges the relative influence of the employees in shaping and developing their healthy living choices. Considering education, they measure the number of diplomas from primary school and upper secondary school but additionally include an indicator on the extent to which pupils can influence school.

It is worth noting that under objective 9, "increased physical activity," they propose as indicator the percentage of the population who walk or cycle in relation to total personal transport. Once again this is a clear example of how success in meeting health targets requires consideration of the close partnership with other non-health sectors, such as transport and city planning. Changes are essential in these areas to facilitate the healthy choices made by individuals.

In summary, there is a wealth of health information collected by different organizations each with a distinct conceptual model of public health. The consideration of health determinants and broader societal factors is apparent in some of the models, although while the inclusion of lifestyle factors and other individual determinants has become more acceptable, the acknowledgment of the influence of upstream factors, that is the social determinants of health, remains a necessity. One conclusion that can be drawn from this section is that there is no shortage of health information gathered in developed countries. We have merely touched upon a few of the many initiatives collecting data relevant to health monitoring, those that we consider more relevant. One can see that in many of the initiatives the indicators chosen reflect mostly health or health-care-related phenomena and a limited inclusion of sociodemographic data. These indicators have limited accountability application for policy makers, in that they do not clearly identify what policies are needed to improve health. Some potentials and pitfalls of single indicators were described already in the first part of this chapter. Nonetheless, some isolated initiatives do strive to include intermediate health determinants and upstream factors, illustrating the link with policies from other sectors. A key challenge is to identify indicators that can be used for accountability in the short term as in many cases socioeconomic or environmental factors may take years to have an effect on health.

Summary Health Indicators: Strengths and Limitations

If innovation in health intelligence for better health governance is to be achieved through the opportune use of indicators, they need to be attractive to policy makers, to the public and to the media. The utility of summary measures of health and well-being is undeniable. In some instances, summary measures that can be used as a way to rank communities, regions, or countries are very attractive to some of the stakeholders; however, the black box appearance of such indicators could be a barrier to use in some advocacy initiatives. Table 6 displays a selection of composite well-being indexes calculated at a national level for international comparison or assessment of national progress. Although the list is by no means exhaustive, we hope to explore the experiences in capturing a more holistic picture of the nation's well-being and to evaluate whether some proposals, either summary indexes or individual indicators included in the indexes, could contribute to the aim of advocating for Health in All Policies.

Although the summary indexes presented have application at different levels of governance, we will highlight the most relevant ones regardless of their application level. Perhaps the most well-known composite indicator is the Human Development Index (HDI) [41] produced yearly for over 91 countries in the world by the United Nations. By combining life expectancy, education, and the gross domestic product (GDP), the HDI has had considerable international impact and has enabled the production of a chart ranking those participating countries. In developed countries, improved sensitivity is achieved through the consideration of additional factors. There is great variation in those factors considered, once again reflecting the values of the institution and the purpose of the index. The Genuine Progress Indicator (GPI) [42], first proposed in 1995 as a substitute for the GDP, captures factors such as family beakdown, income distribution, or changes in leisure time, hoping to portray a more honest picture of the nation's well-being. The Social and Cultural planning Office (SCP) of the Netherlands Living Conditions Index [48] give a very high weight to leisure time with three of their eight sub-indices being leisure activity, sport activity, and holiday activity.

Any one of the summary indexes depicted in Table 6 has advantages and limitations; however, for advocacy purposes, perhaps the most relevant work is that carried out by the Fordham Institute of Innovation in Social Policy. They have calculated the Social Health Index for the USA since 1990 and shown that as the GDP of the USA continually rises, this is not met by a similar increase in the social health of the nation [50, 52]. A closer look at the indicators they have chosen reveals that in addition to classical health indicators such as infant mortality, they include various social factors pertinent to health at distinct life stages. By estimating high school drop outs (early school leavers), they have an education indicator which can change on a monthly basis and can easily be evaluated in different subgroups, such as residential areas, and give key information on inequalities. The school drop-out rate is an indirect measure of education, and education is often the key determinant underlying most socioeconomic analyses of health outcomes [53]. However, the pathways by which education, and more precisely dropping out of high school, may affect health, are numerous, and may function though distinct determinants later in life such as income level, health literacy, psychosocial support network, etc. [54–57].

Some indicators that monitor educational functioning are sensitive in the short-medium term, yet are representative of long-term health effects and closely linked to non-health policies. These same features are shared by other component indicators of the Social Health Index (child poverty, teenage suicide rates, etc.), and we feel that this kind of data should be included in the set of indicators for public health monitoring.

Returning to summary indexes, none of the proposals match perfectly in what would be an ideal summary index suitable for enhancing the visibility of the health

Table 6 Indices measuring the well-being of the Nation(s)

Summary indicator	Reporting body	Components: indicators	Year started	Countries
Human Development Index (HDI) [41]	United Nations	Index calculated on 3 dimensions: 1. Life expectancy at birth 2. Education (2/3 adult literacy : 1/3 school enrolment statistics) 3. GDP	1990	91 countries
Genuine Progress Indicador (GPI) [42]	Redefining Progress (US based public policy think tank), California, USA	Adjusts GDP incorporating: • Crime and family breakdown • Household and volunteer work • Income distribution • Resource depletion • Pollution • Long-term environmental damage • Changes in leisure time • Defensive expenditures • Life span of consumer durables and public infrastructure • Dependence on foreign assets	1995	Initially USA only. Adopted by various others.
Quality of Life Index (QOL) [43]	Diener, Department of Psychology, University of Illinois	7 indicators: • Purchasing power • Homicide rate • Fulfilment of basic physical needs • Suicide rate • Literacy rate • Gross human rights violations • Deforestation	1995	101 countries

Table 6 (continued)

Summary indicator	Reporting body	Components: indicators	Year started	Countries
The Advanced QOL Index (to assess QOL in highly industrialized nations)		7 Indicators: • Physicians per capita • Savings rate • Per capita income • Subjective well-being • Percent attending college • Income equality • Environmental treaties signed		
Mother's Index [44]	Save the Children (Report: *The state of the world mothers*)	Index composed of 10 indicators: 6 Women's indicators • Maternal mortality • % Woman using modern contraception • % Births attended by trained personnel • % Pregnant women with anaemia • Adult female literacy • Participation of women in national government 4 Children indicators • Infant mortality • Gross primary enrolment ratio • % Population with access to safe water • % <5 years with moderate/severe nutritional wasting	2000	105 countries

Table 6 (continued)

Summary indicator	Reporting body	Components: indicators	Year started	Countries
Index of Human Progress (IHP) [45]	Fraser Institute, Vancouver, British Columbia, Canada	Health: • Life expectancy • Infant mortality • <5 years mortality • Adult mortality Education: • Literacy • Combined enrolment ratio Technology: • No. of televisions per 1000 • No. of radios per 1000 • Telephone service GDP	2001 published results from 1975–1999	128 countries
Weighted Index of Social Progress (WISP) [46]	University of Pennsylvania	40 indicators in 10 sub-indices: • Education • Health status • Woman status • Defence effort • Economic • Demographic • Environment • Social chaos • Cultural diversity • Welfare effort	1984 (revised 1997)	160 countries
Human Well-Being Index (HWI) [47]	Prescott-Allan (with support of IUCN –The World Conservation Union and	36 indicators in 5 sub-indices: • Health and population • Wealth	2003 publication: *The Well-being of Nations*	180 countries

Table 6 (continued)

Summary indicator	Reporting body	Components: indicators	Year started	Countries
	the International Development Research Centre (IDRC))	• Knowledge and culture • Community • Equity		
Living Conditions Index (LCI) [48]	Social and Cultural Planning Office (SCP), Netherlands	Sub-indices include: • Housing • Health • Purchasing power • Leisure activities • Mobility • Social participation • Sport activity • Holiday activity	1974 (updated and revised 1997)	15 member states of the EU 1995–2001
Index of Individual Living Conditions [49]	ZUMA – Centre for Survey Research and Methodology, Mannheim, Germany	Seven sub-indices: • Income/standard of living • Housing • Housing area • Education • Health • Social relations • Work	1995	15 member states of the EU 1995–2001
Fordham Social Health Index [50]	Fordham University Institute for Innovation in Social Policy	16 Indicators in 5 domains • Children: (Infant mortality, Child abuse, Child poverty) • Youth: (Teenage suicide, Teenage drug abuse, High school dropouts)	1987	USA

Table 6 (continued)

Summary indicator	Reporting body	Components: indicators	Year started	Countries
		• Adults: (Unemployment, Average weekly wages, Health insurance coverage) • Aging: (Poverty among those aged 65 and and over, Out-of-pocket health costs among those aged 65 and over • All ages: (Homicides, Alcohol-related traffic fatalities, Food stamp coverage, Access to affordable housing, Income inequality)		
Canadian Index of Well-being (CIW) [51]	Atkinson Foundation, Toronto, Canada	Seven domains: • Living standards • Time allocation • Healthy populations • Ecosystem health • Educated populace • Community vitality • Civic engagement	Currently being developed	Canada

effects of non-health policies and in evaluating general progress or macro-policies. An ideal summary measure should be close to the macroeconomic indexes reported monthly, such as inflation of consumer prices. If we had a monthly reported index of health and well-being that took in measures of social health and other health-related features, decision makers would pay more attention to those policies that have indirect effects on health. The Social Health Index meets some of the aspects of an ideal index, but data availability precludes its regular estimation and some of its components are not sensitive to medium-short-term changes.

In conclusion, we already have several proposals of summary health indexes, yet none of them fit the requirements for use in achieving high visibility for the health effects of non-health policies. Nevertheless, the work done so far is an apt starting point that with further research could allow the availability of such a summary index to be tested as an advocacy tool. Most of the work needed refers to the component indicators that are included in the summary index. On the other hand, a summary index could be useful in general advocacy for health in other policies but not appropriate in promoting specific policies or for influencing particular decision makers at lower levels. Summary indexes do not indicate who is accountable for the results nor their specific policy implications. In the next sections, we shall consider comparative risk assessment and health impact assessment.

Comparative Risk Assessment

A major advance in the management of health information for the improvement of population health was the launch of comparative risk assessment. This approach permits the quantification of the health effects (mortality, morbidity, disability) which can be causally attributed to major risk factors. The most comprehensive work on population attributable risk is the Comparative Risk Assessment Global Burden of Disease (GBD) study 2000 [58] (Box 4). The approach chosen by the authors of this study is widely accepted and used extensively by International Health Institutions. Estimates are published yearly in the World Health Organization Report.

Box 4. The Global Burden of Disease Project

The WHO Global Burden of Disease (GBD) project has updated the original Global Burden of Disease Study carried out by Murray and Lopez for the year 1990.

The WHO GBD project draws on a wide range of data sources to develop internally consistent estimates of incidence, health state prevalence, severity and duration, and mortality for over 130 major causes, for WHO Member States and for sub-regions of the world, for the years 2000 and beyond.

WHO program participation in the development and finalization of these estimates ensures that estimates reflect all information and knowledge available to

WHO. The WHO is now undertaking a new assessment of the Global Burden of Disease for the year 2004.
    Broadly, the GBD provides comprehensive estimates of the disease burden at a global, regional and national level that can be attributed to a variety of known risk factors.

This excerpt is taken directly from the WHO website. For further information can be obtained from: www.who.int/healthinfo/bodabout/en/index.html

Key Points:

- The GBD uses disability adjusted life years (DALY) to quantify the burden of disease.
- One DALY can be thought of as one year of 'healthy' life lost through premature death, poor health or disability.
- The burden of disease can be considered a measurement of the gap between current health status and an ideal situation where everyone lives into old age free of disease and disability.
- The GBD calculates the DALYS that would be saved if each risk was reduced to a theoretical minimum.

The GBD objective was to assess the impact at a population level of various proximal risk factors (underweight, blood pressure, unsafe sex, cholesterol, alcohol, etc.), environmental factors (unsafe water, outdoor air pollution, etc.), or occupational factors (noise, injury risk, etc). The GDB poses the question, "of the entire disease burden in this population, how much could be caused by this risk?" The initial project involved 26 expert groups carrying out an extensive review of all available evidence to obtain comprehensive estimates of risk factor prevalence and effects. The outcome is expressed in disability adjusted life years (DALYS), representing the number of years in disability-free health that would be saved if exposure to each risk was reduced to the theoretical minimum level. According to their results, the single leading cause of health loss globally is childhood underweight, causing the loss of 138 million DALYS, which corresponds to 9.5% of world health loss.

This study represented a major innovation in health information management because it revealed that a large proportion of global health loss can be attributed to a relatively small number of factors. This, with the fact that a disproportionately small amount of resources is directed towards reducing these risk factors, is an important consideration in health governance. Nonetheless, when considering the information needs of decision makers, some aspects of the study leave room for further development.

Although calculations are made separately for geographical region, sex, and age group, the GDB study falls short of stratifying data by socioeconomic status, ethnic group, or other categories related to upstream determinants. Consequently, it is difficult to identify where the inequalities lie and on what groups interventions should focus in order to achieve greatest health benefits. In developed regions the leading cause of loss of healthy life, contributing to mainly noncommunicable diseases, are tobacco, high blood pressure, alcohol, high cholesterol, and high BMI. Notice that all five of these risk factors are linked to individual health behaviors. There is little consideration of the fact that the role of any single risk factor is likely to be affected by structural determinants such as education, income, social class, gender, and ethnic group, and intermediary social determinants such as material circumstances, psychosocial circumstances, biological factors, and the health system itself [34]. Moreover, most of the mentioned determinants exert their critical and cumulative effects throughout the life course.

It has been acknowledged that while the measurement of aggregate health outcomes and individual risk factors clearly satisfy the purpose of describing the population health status and identifying important health risks, when it comes to attributing cause, or the evaluation of policies, their use is limited because they provide no insight into the processes involved in their modification [59]. Despite criticism, we mention the GBD study in this section as we feel that is a powerful innovation in the evolution of health information management. Quantifying the disease burden attributable to a variety of risk factors or health determinants is useful in assessing priorities and setting health targets. The approach used in this study and other comparative risk assessments may prove useful in our purposes of reorganizing health information for better governance, as we shall discuss later in the chapter.

Health Impact Assessment

Health Impact Assessment (HIA) (Box 5) is a tool designed to support the health implications in decision making at all political and administrative levels. The procedures and methods of HIA are universally applicable, and as such can be applied to proposals from any sector in order to minimize detrimental effects and maximize benefits on population health.

Box 5. Health Impact Assessment

Health impact assessment (HIA) developed in response to the universal acknowledgement that policies or programs from other sectors can have a considerable influence on health.

It calls for the evaluation and explicit consideration of potential health impacts caused by any new public policy or community program to aid decision maker and in order to mitigate the negative and maximize the positive impacts.

In the WHO Regional office for Europe and European Centre for Health Policy Gothenburg consensus paper HIA is defined as

*A combination of procedures, methods and tools by which a policy, programme or
project may be judged as to its potential effects on the health of a population, and
the distribution of those effects within the population*[60]

Further information on HIA and links can be obtained from the following
website: www.who.int/hia/en/

Key Points

- HIA should be multidisciplinary, intersectoral, and participatory.
- Both quantitative and qualitative types of evidence should be considered.
- The process of HIA comprises the following stages [61]:

  o *Screening* (a systematic approach aimed to identify proposals for which
    a HIA would be useful)
  o *Scoping* (identification of the populations and communities affected, the
    potential health impacts and selection of the appropriate methods for the
    HIA)
  o *Appraisal or risk assessment* (identification and assessment of positive
    and negative health impacts)
  o Preparation of report and recommendations
  o Submission of report and recommendations to decision makers
  o Monitoring and evaluation

HIA differs from comprehensive risk assessment in that it does not attempt to
combine the different outcomes in a single metric such as DALYS, but rather to consider all possible health outcomes though a series of evidence-based assumptions. In
essence, an HIA attempts to show all plausible pathways by which a certain policy
may affect health and to quantify all health effects, positive and adverse. As such,
the results from an HIA may include a variety of outcomes in addition to mortality
and morbidity estimates, some of which may not be properly quantified in summary
health indexes such as possible increase in anxiety.

The proponents of HiAP give an exceptional role to health impact assessment
and foresee that its application will promote the inclusion of health as an effect of
any policy. The current level of implementation of HIA in Europe varies [62], and
it has been acknowledged that in many cases it is more common at the local rather
than a national level. In fact its application is particularly opportune at local level
where, through network governance, as described by Warner in his chapter, the barriers for collaboration across sectors and for HIA implementation can be overcome.
In practice organizations may be dissuaded from carrying out a HIA due to the
belief that it is time-consuming and requires specialist knowledge and uncertainty
on how to begin. There is some debate about institutionalizing HIA in Europe. Institutionalizing refers to the systematic integration of the approach as part of the rules

and procedures involved in policy appraisal. While institutionalizing HIA would increase acceptability and use, the concern is that it may restrict the scope for political advocacy since it would require the impartiality of the HIA practitioner [63, 64]. A key aspect of HIA is stakeholder participation, involving the people affected by, or who have an interest in, the decision. One of the principles of new health governance –"health policy and target initiatives can arise at any point in the system and be initiated by any actor" [2] – is especially applicable to HIA.

A central issue in developing HIA is determining which actors produce and provide the relevant data to perform the assessment. Although we hold that the public health force should engage in active advocacy to extend HIA implementation, the involved sectors are who should lead the assessment or, at least, the process could be jointly developed between sectors. Anyway, particular attention should be paid to the coordinative role and its special features in network governance (See Chapter 5: Health in All Policies at the local level. Governance through "virtual reorganization by design")

An HIA carried out to assess the public health benefits of reducing air pollution in the Barcelona metropolitan area found that in addition to approximately 3500 fewer annual deaths (520 of which are due to short term exposure), reducing current levels of air pollution to the WHO standards would result in an annual reduction of 1800 hospital admissions for cardiorespiratory diseases, 5100 cases of chronic bronchitis symptoms among adults, 31,100 cases of acute bronchitis among children, and 54,000 asthma attacks among children and adults [63].

The example of outdoor air pollution could present an over-simplification of the procedures involved in HIA. While the relative health benefits due to improved air quality are well accepted, the health effect of other policies is less covered in the research agenda and this is a limitation for evidence based HIA. Nevertheless the potential for HIA is huge and its increasing popularity should in itself advocate for more focus on this area through highlighting where deficits lie.

We mention HIA here as we believe it illustrates another important advance in health intelligence, promoting a multidisciplinary responsibility for the protection of population health. Furthermore, in this section we have attempted to identify health information which clearly provides a link to specific policies and HIA is designed explicitly for this purpose. In the final part of this chapter we shall discuss how we believe HIA should be taken a step further for better governance.

Part III: Outlook: How Can We Meet the Expectations of Intelligence for Better Governance?

Requirements of Useful Indicators

When previously analyzing the component indicators of the Social Health Index, we advanced some of the qualities that single health indicators require in order to be useful for advocacy for Health in All Policies. The indicator must be *illustrative* of the link with policies including those non-health policies. There is a need for *immediacy*, meaning that the indicator is able to reflect changes incurred in the short or medium term. The final characteristic is *feasibility*, that the data required is available or can feasibly be obtained. The ability to use existing data available in the majority of administrative areas and population groups is considered critical for developing indicators. An additional feature required is that the indicator monitors a policy with relevant health impact. Frequency, severity of the health effect, economic impact, emergent status of the condition, and level of public concern are among the standard criteria for assessment of public health relevance. As we wish to stress the potential for advocacy, public concern, media attractiveness, and decision-maker susceptibility become essential criteria.

Usual requirements of indicators, mainly validity, are pertinent but we will not comment on this feature as it has been extensively considered in documents on public health surveillance. For the purposes of advocacy, a key quality is immediacy. When considering upstream health determinants, immediacy is of utmost relevance because the effects on health caused by broader societal factors such as education may take years to incur [53, 57]. An attractive indicator should provide an indication of current changes in order to aid decision making and the setting up of timely interventions. Illustrating the link to non-health policies may pose a challenge. We propose that it may require the monitoring of determinants which have an established relationship with health, rather than monitoring the health outcome itself.

Indicators Addressing the Social Determinants of Health

The case of social conditions in childhood and youth, whose relevant effects last over the life course, is a paradigm of social exposures with long latency periods. Evidence is accumulating on the enormous potential deleterious health effects of disadvantaged social conditions during childhood and youth. Low socioeconomic characteristics of family of origin is associated with higher morbidity and mortality in adulthood: those with low childhood socioeconomic status have an increased mortality and morbidity risk of chronic diseases such as stroke, cardiovascular disease or depression, low functional status in middle life, and worse self-rated health. In addition to living conditions in the parental home, youth education trajectories, and, to a minor degree, employment and marital trajectories have a relevant effect on social class differences in total mortality among men in their middle adulthood [54].

That conditions in these periods of life are critical is common knowledge; however, their health effects over the whole life course are rarely known and even unfamiliar to many health professionals. Promoting educational and other socioeconomic policies in critical periods like reproduction, childhood, and youth is a huge health investment. The aim is to reduce inequalities and assure a minimum of material and social conditions that prevent unhealthy trajectories in future life. Although, apart from health, there are other ethical bases to ensure a minimum level of social conditions in early life periods, the fact is that disadvantaged backgrounds are common in developed countries and are a major contributor to adult health disparities.

Putting health in the promotion of these policies could be a way of strengthening their implementation.

Increasing the number of indicators of early life social conditions in the public health surveillance set is a first step in giving relevance to the connection of these conditions and health. Indicators such as those included in the Social Health Index (child poverty, teenage suicide, high-school drop outs) together with other indicators more clearly linked to the health domain, such as low birth-weight, teenage pregnancy, etc., should be highlighted in the monitoring of health. Other very specific indicators such as teenage abortion rates could play a relevant role if their values turn out to show a good correlation with early social indicators (high school attainment, parental conditions, etc.) and other health-related issues. We acknowledge the difficulties in tracing the health affects related to early life interventions and the influences of education.

Indicators of classical risk factors such as obesity, physical activity or fruit and vegetable consumption are already included in usual public health surveillance systems and some of them take up substantial space in usual institutional health reports. Many of the interventions aimed to change prevalence of these factors depend on non-health policies. An opportune way to frame the information in order to favor these policies would be the design of indicators that account for the density of policies linked to the risk factors. We already mentioned in Box 1 the need to assess the density of policies that are guided under the principles of Health in All Policies, which is also a proposal mentioned in an accompanying document to the White Paper, Together for Health of the European Union [65]. A constant difficulty in designing such indicators is the lack of research on effective policies; for example, a review of population interventions on nutrition did not find the assessment of any policy [66]. However, for many of the relevant risk factors, there are enough policies that, if not implemented, are at least recommended and can be quantified and monitored. Pilot projects in setting up this type of indicator could demonstrate their feasibility and encourage their use.

Health impacts of environmental factors are among the most commonly studied. For some exposures, the causal framework is reasonably complete and there are sufficient data on how policy actions impact the framework (e.g., lead exposure) [67]. In this case, the available knowledge on quantitative information allows not only the estimation of the disease burden caused by environmental exposure but also a prediction of health gains according to policy actions. Some environmental indicators are usually included in public health surveillance reports, specifically those that measure outdoor air pollution such as particulate matter (PM). Extensive work has been carried out to assess the burden of disease attributable to environmental factors [68–71] as well as the potential impact of a series of policies aimed at tackling the sources of environmental exposures. Integrating health in environmental policies can be enhanced at lower decision levels by opportune use of available information.

As shown in next section, we can convert the results of burden of disease attributable to environmental factors together with health impact assessments into policy indicators that express the yearly or monthly healthy life years that would be gained through an individual policy if it were implemented. Information regarding the impact on health of some policies on physical built environment is not as complete as that available on environmental exposures to toxic contaminants. Nevertheless, a growing number of research reports show solid association between several results of urban planning policies and health-related lifestyles such as physical activity [72–75]. This gives the opportunity to create intermediate indicators such as density of green zones. As with the previous indicators considered in this section, the best way of framing the available information is by linking the individual policy with the health outcome.

Single indicators on other health determinants and related policies can also be generated in order to facilitate intersectoral action. Opportune indicators could be a key tool in promoting polices on working conditions, unemployment or gender inequalities, among others, that could improve the population health. In summary, in all non-health policy sectors where enough knowledge is available on the causal pathways between determinants and health outcomes as well as on the effect of policies on these determinants, there is an opportunity to create indicators as a means of advocating for the integration of health in other policies. Some of the indicators discussed could be added in a new summary index as those previously described. Other measurements could be part of routine public health surveillance as proposed for early life conditions. Finally, some of the indicators can be applied solely in advocacy.

In all cases, actions should be taken to ensure that all information on health determinants – from individual determinants to structural determinants – and health outcomes is provided for relevant socioeconomic strata. Socioeconomic variables at all levels – from the geographical area to the individual – must be at the core of health information since interventions and policies to reduce health inequities are the top priority of non-health policies.

Reframing Health Information for Better Governance

Estimating the disease burden attributable to risk factors, as in the aforementioned global burden of disease study (Box 4), can be very informative and is an appreciable step in enhancing health information. It has been suggested that together with information on the costs of interventions, their effectiveness, and the socioeconomic context, such knowledge provides a rational basis for policy setting. However, it is remarkable that the attribution of disease is made not to the root underlying causes of disease but to proximal causes that do not clearly indicate the needed policies. We propose that these calculations be taken a step further.

Attributing 7.4% of all health loss in developed countries to high BMI is not informative enough for policy makers. A calculation of health loss that could be avoided by adoption of an intervention proven to be successful in reducing the BMI could be used in promoting such policy. Framing the information in this way has clear policy implications and could indicate who or which institution is accountable for implementing the effective policy. This indicator (the DALYS potentially

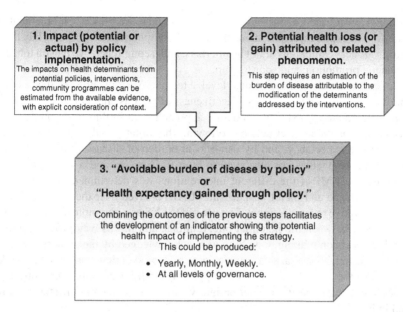

Fig. 1 Creating innovative indicators which offer **transparency** and **accountability** to decision makers

saved or healthy life years gained by policy implementation) can offer policy makers information that is transparent and easily applicable. The indicator proposed can be estimated for *all levels of decision making* and at *regular time intervals*, when data are available. These are paramount qualities for the use of the indicator in advocacy. This possibility is illustrated in Fig. 1.

Calculating DALYS attributable to new policies is often a requirement for cost-effectiveness analysis and extending the GBD risk estimates to potential policies is an approach that has already been covered by some studies of larger populations. It has been predicted that legislation to decrease salt content in processed foods and appropriate labelling could lead to a reduction in 13,000 DALYS over 10 years in subset of European countries [76]. Similarly, health education through mass media campaigns could save 12,000 DALYS in the same time period. Another study estimates the health benefits attributable to a reduction in salt intake of 15% [77] (theoretically obtained through the voluntary reduction in the salt content of processed foods and condiments by manufacturers, and a sustained mass-media campaign aimed at encouraging dietary change within households and communities). By estimating the relationship between sodium intake and change in systolic blood pressure and then applying the risk attributable to high systolic blood pressure from the GBD study, the authors calculate that 8.5 million deaths could be averted in the 23 low-middle income countries studied over 10 years. In a similar manner they calculate that 5.5 million deaths could be averted over the 10-year period by the adoption of a selection of the interventions recommended by the WHO framework convention on tobacco control (FCTC): namely, increased taxes, enforcement of smoke-free workplaces, requirements for FCTC-compliant packaging and labelling, public awareness campaigns about health risks, and a comprehensive ban on tobacco advertising, promotion, and sponsorship.

In a similar manner, but at national level, a team in Australia presented an assessment of the health benefit and cost effectiveness of various childhood or adolescent obesity interventions [78]. The modeling approach used in this study predicts the likely health intervention effects by following the target populations though their remaining life expectancy, and by using local burden of disease estimates to take into account the health risks attributed to high BMI by sex and 5-year age group. The impact on BMI of the different interventions was determined using the best available evidence and then translated into DALYS saved over the child's lifetime using comparative risk assessment. The use of DALYS as a common outcome allows a comparison between the potential interventions, and in this way provides a useful tool for decision making. One limitation acknowledged by the authors is that in order to make a fair comparison between potential interventions, one must also take into account the strength of evidence supporting each intervention. An outline of one of the potential obesity prevention interventions considered in the study can be found in Fig. 2.

This project received criticism for the major assumption that any health effect achieved in the intervention group would be maintained into adult life, as this assumption was the basis for translation into DALYS [79]. In response to this point it may be possible to integrate the recent advances in prediction seen in the UK Foresight report on tackling obesity [80]. In this modeling exercise the authors are able to predict reliably future trends in obesity, owing to close inspection of 12 years of

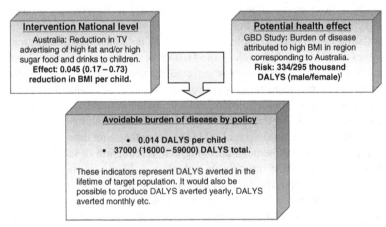

Fig. 2 Avoidable burden of disease attributable to obesity through policy on publicity.
[†]The figures reported here come from the 2000 GBD study and consequently reflect the DALYS averted should the risk "high BMI" be reduced to a theoretical minimum of 21. Together with local burden of disease estimates, it is possible to extrapolate the potential impact of the observed intervention effect in the study population.

data from England's health survey and the revelation that obesity trends in England follow "meticulous order and consistency." In brief, they use two computer-based prediction models: the first was used to process the information from the health survey and construct a model predicting the likely future growth of the population; the second is a microsimulation of obesity growth, capable of statistically quantifying both recent history and future changes in obesity levels based on the results from the first program. In the study, the microsimulation models the population of England from the mid-1990s to the end of the 21st century. Using the current age, gender and disease distributions, the authors predict the obesity-related disease and death rates. Similarly, by anticipating the consequences of interventions on BMI prevalence by age, gender, and year, they were able to simulate the effects on predicted obesity related morbidity and mortality and therefore explore how their levels would develop following such interventions.

A key strength of this foresight study is that the computer-generated prediction models are flexible and easy to use. They can be modified to consider additional parameters such as ethnicity or socioeconomic status. Similarly, the user can input baseline population characteristics and specify the risk factors associated with obesity that they wish to be considered. In addition, and perhaps the most relevant for our purposes is that among potential uses, the microsimulation has the capability of modelling for user-specifiable interventions and effects. In this way, the Foresight project offers a tool capable of estimating the future impact on health of any obesity intervention (provided evidence of its effects on BMI). These methods could be applied to other health situations and populations thereby providing means by which to consider the potential long-term health effects of current interventions from any sector. Consequently, we feel that it is a major innovation in health intelligence for better governance.

We acknowledge that any indicator that links potential non-health policies with health outcomes has a series of limitations. On the one hand, there are the limitations of the burden of disease estimations already discussed elsewhere [81, 82]. On the other hand, there are the limitations themselves of assessing the effects of policies on health determinants and the temporal frame of the effects.

The temporal frame limitation refers to the fact that for interventions with long-term health outcomes, an indicator of present burden of disease attributed to any policy on determinants of health will render very low or null values. This phenomenon is relevant to most policies but with considerable variations. For instance, not all benefits of policies aimed at improving air quality will be detectable in the first year, but it has been estimated that one could expect 40% of the total annual death benefits to materialize within the first year [83]. For interventions in early life, the situation is quite the inverse, as health benefits need many years, often decades, to become evident. Consider, for example, interventions aimed at increasing fruit and vegetable intake carried out in elementary schools which have been shown to increase consumption by 30–35 g per day [84]. It is reasonable to assume that eating habits and behaviors adopted at this age may affect determinants in later life and the health effects may be quite substantial. In addition morbidity caused by low fruit and vegetable intake will function through diverse pathways such as disorders associated with obesity, which in themselves are not immediate. Due to the latency of these health effects, loss of healthy life attributable to lack of fruit and vegetable in-take is rarely detected in elementary school children, as illustrated by stratification of the GBD project by age [85]. Accordingly, indicators of avoidable burden of disease by policies should be time framed. Developments and advances in prediction methodology, such as those seen in the Foresight study, would be one way to consider the likely future trends.

Another key limitation of this approach is the shortage of information. The feasibility of these indicators relies on evidence of the effects of interventions on those determinants of health and risk factors with an established health effect. While the health effect of numerous different risk factors is an active area of research, the benefits obtained from policies is more difficult to ascertain. Additionally research on upstream health determinants that provide risk estimations to calculate the attributable burden is scarce. Similarly, while the effects of specific health interventions aimed at reducing risk factors may be feasibly obtained, discerning the consequences of non-health policies may prove challenging due to lack of research.

So far, some of the examples discussed refer to policies which have as their main objective to reduce certain health risks or determinants. Our proposal is that this type of tool should be extended to interventions from other sectors not necessarily aimed specifically at tackling health risks. As we have discussed in this chapter, the effects of such policies is often very difficult to ascertain due to multiple and complex pathways. To tackle these challenges, we propose that HIA (Box 5) be used to account for diverse pathways by which non-health policies may affect health. Environmental air pollution offers a good example as, although not all health benefits would be detectable immediately, the strategies to reduce air pollution have been shown to produce immediate and sustained improvements in air quality. The immediate health benefits such as fewer cases of acute bronchitis in children or fewer hospital admissions for cardiorespiratory disease would be observed in parallel with improvements in air quality. Moreover, a significant proportion of the total annual death benefits reduction in mortality would materialize in the first year as previously mentioned [86]. Monitoring those indicators sensitive to improvements in air quality in the short term could be used to monitor progress and accountability for policy makers and stakeholders.

Our model applied here would use the outcomes of current HIA projects to provide indicators of health loss or gain resulting from individual policies. These indicators are not limited to health expectancy estimates measured in DALYS, but can produce a series of more concrete outcomes, such as the number of hospital admissions or number of childhood asthma cases that could be avoided by implementation of a certain traffic policy (Fig. 3). In this way the results from current HIA provide indicators offering transparency for decision makers and, for the purposes of advocacy, can be calculated monthly by interest groups to illustrate the mortality or morbidity that has not been avoided each month due to failure to adopt the policy or inaction by the policy maker. Innovation in health policy requires an expansion of the current use of HIA. As well as a policy appraisal process it should also be used by

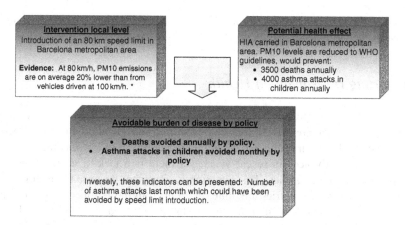

Fig. 3 Avoidable burden of disease through a traffic calming scheme in Barcelona
*In order to product this indicator, a reliable estimate of the expected PM10 effect is required.

any stakeholders in an effort to produce indicators of "avoidable burden of disease by policy" and advocate for policy change. HIA as described here, instead of seeking to convince policy makers of its advantages, represents a more proactive approach.

In summary, the estimation of disease burden attributable to several risk factors at a multinational scale contributes to a call for action in order to control the causes of the relevant public health problems. The fact that inequity and that the intermediary and structural causes (which include policies) are frequently omitted in these estimations could incline the preventive response towards proximal risks factors and medical approaches. The integration of non-health policies in general preventive strategies requires the estimation of the burden of disease attributed to several factors in smaller populations (cities, school districts, neighborhoods, etc.) and development of the avoidable burden through policies that match the same population level. We hold that figures of this kind could be calculated and would represent relevant indicators at all levels of decision making, from small institutional communities such as schools or workplaces, to the regional or national level. Developing population-specific "avoidable burden by policy indicators" provides a useful tool in advocacy and provides policy makers with the kind of information which is relevant to their policy context. For example, a local council is more likely to act on the information delivered if it illustrates that facilitating alternative methods of transport to work, through the provision of cycle paths, could save X health loss in their district, rather than if it informs them of the global health loss attributable to physical inactivity. In summary, the ability to calculate these indicators at all levels of decision making provide us with a very appealing advocacy tool.

The second important point, already advanced, is that these indicators can be produced at regular intervals as part of the public health surveillance effort or by the relevant interest groups. For the purposes of advocacy and moving health considerations further up the political agenda, this is very powerful. If the proposed indicators that show the avoidable health burden by policy can be produced weekly, monthly, or yearly, the public and media impact could be greatly enhanced.

Supporting Investment on Health

Finally, and importantly for advocating this approach, is the need to illustrate the role of health as a major driving force for economic and social productivity. Recognizing the link between health and economic development in low-income countries has seen major advances in recent years, yet there is a lack of attention paid to this process in rich countries. This situation is important because the health problems in high-income countries are quite different from those affecting low-income countries. The morbidity in high-income countries is predominantly due to health problems which require complex interventions. It is therefore harder to illustrate the benefits obtained from investments in health. The relative lack of research in this area, and the gaps that exist in knowledge of this process are now being increasingly recognized [87]. The situation in high-income countries is often limited to cost of illness studies, which are usually carried out for the purposes of identifying the economic burden of illness rather than defending health investment as an economic driving force.

Furthermore, some of the pathways by which health can affect economic competitively are complex. Consider, for example, interventions to promote good health in childhood. Children in better health have enhanced cognitive functions and show reduced school absenteeism. Hence, it is safe to assume that children with better health can be expected to attain a higher level of education and therefore be more productive in the future [87]. Producing evidence of such a link is a difficult task and shares the same limitations as the identification of the health impact of distal health determinants.

In summary, information accounting for the effects of health on economic productivity and illustrating the potential benefits derived from health investment is much needed. Isolated studies suggest that workplace health promotion programs can produce sizeable changes in health risks and productivity within the workplace [88]. Unfortunately, although most corporate decision makers accept the intuitive link between employee health and productivity, there is a barrier in addressing the implications of such a link. Employers may be less willing to invest in employee health, due to a lack of clear and quantifiable evidence. Decision makers need to know exactly how much health improvement is required to improve productivity and in turn exactly how much improvement in productivity should they expect from their investment [89]. Once again, information or evidence needs to be framed and placed in the appropriate context, before decision makers are likely to act upon it. For our purposes of identifying potential for innovation in the management of health information, it is necessary to highlight the need for development in this area. Accessible information and implementing research findings will reinforce the opinion that protecting health can have important consequences on realizing the goals of other sectors.

Conclusions

We have shown in this chapter that there are many different data collection efforts and a great wealth of information gathered. Among them, innovations worth mentioning are the Burden of Disease Project and Health Impact Assessment. Health intelligence for better governance requires reorganizing and repackaging this information. New and innovative ways of framing health information are needed, particularly if we wish to convince non-health sectors of the relevance of health in their policies.

We propose the regular production of indicators which clearly account for the health effect of specific policies. Reporting health loss or gain attributable to specific policies could be successful in promoting health as an important consideration in all policies. Providing indicators of health loss or gain attributable to policy action clearly links health outcomes with policy. Predicting avoidable disease or mortality that has not been avoided due to failure to adopt a certain policy would have enormous potential as a tool for advocacy. The relevant points of our proposal are:

- Increased surveillance of the social determinants of health.
- Production of indicators of health gains through specific policies.
- Development of health impact assessment in a proactive manner to avoid policy inaction.
- Linkage of health gains with other societal attainments.

We have discussed at length how to develop the indicators on health gains through policy and we feel that in the future adequate research can provide the relevant knowledge base for better shaping the proposal. More and better evidence is needed to advance in the four aspects considered and special attention should be paid to developing the economic bases for financing the policies on social determinants of health. There is a clear necessity for proposals that produce information on the effects of health investment in economic and social domains. Furthermore, information is needed to strengthen the links and increase the validity of current health impact assessments. Further research is clearly needed; however, we would also like to stress the following axes that are transversal to our proposals:

- Relevant policy linked indicators should be produced at *every governance level*, and each governance level should apply the approach that most appropriate to its environment.
- Policies themselves are relevant health determinants and outcomes of governance. *Policy density and trends* should be included in health information management.
- Health information management should consider the context. Indicators such as "health expectancy gained through policy" must take into account *inequalities*

(by socioeconomic level, gender, residence, ethnicity, and so on) in a manner that directs policies to those in society that need more attention.

– Any health information proposal must favor *accountability* by those sectors, governmental or otherwise, of the decisions which can make people healthier.

– Health information should be produced and framed to assure high *visibility of health and well-being* and in a way that can be understood by the public (*transparency*), and that motivates their participation in public issues related to health.

– Innovations in health information must contribute to a strengthened public health advocacy. *Advocacy* is needed to develop Health in All Policies, to increase accountability and transparency and to engage all interest groups in new health governance.

We have shown how innovation in health information contributes to good health governance. We want to underline that health reporting should be integrated in the policy process and not be an obstacle to policy implementation. Insufficient evidence should stimulate policy innovation rather than merely more research. Indeed we need to develop implementation science [90] integrating a multidisciplinary systematic approach to address the gap between innovations in health and policy. If evaluation of complex social programs is needed, policy implementation and health intelligence should be combined in order to increase evidence and provide illustrative models. Researchers and public health professionals must participate in the actions of the so-called "third community" [91], in bridging the gap between research and policy. This process involves tailoring information to the policy context and we believe our proposals for indicators of health gain through policy could be one way to achieve this.

References

1. Marinker M, editor. Targets in Europe. Polity, Progress and Promise. London: BMJ Books; 2002.
2. Kickbusch I. Perspectives in health governance in the 21st century. In: Marinker M, editor. Targets in Europe. Polity, Progress and Promise. London: BMJ Books; 2002. p. 206–29.
3. Marinker M. Health policy and the constructive conversationalist. In: Marinker M, editor. Constructive Conversations About Health. Policy and Values. Oxon: Radcliffe Publishining Ltd; 2006. p. 1–16.
4. Carlsson P, Garpenby P. Democracy. In: arinker M, editor. Constructive Conversations About Health. Policy and Values. Oxon: Radcliffe Publishing Ltd; 2006. p. 63–74.
5. World Health Organisation. Healthy Cities Around the World: An Overview of the Healthy Cities Movement in the Six WHO Regions. Published on the Occasion of the 2003 International Healthy Cities Conference, Belfast, Northern Ireland, United Kingdom, 19–22 October 2003. Copenhagen, Denmark: WHO Regional Office; 2003.
6. Ottawa Charter for Health Promotion. In: Health Promotion. Vol. 1. Geneva: World Health Organization; 1986. p. iii–v.
7. Rose G. The Strategy of Preventive Medicine. Oxford, England: Oxford University Press Inc; 1992.
8. WHO. Second International Conference on Health Promotion. Adelaide Recommendations on Healthy Public Policy [Online], 1988 [cited 15th Mar 2008]. Available from: www.who.int/healthpromotion/conferences/previous/adelaide/en/index.html

9. Berkman LF, Kawachi I, editors. Social Epidemiology. New York: Oxford University Press; 2000.
10. Kawachi I, Kennedy BP, Wilkinson RG, editors. The Society and Population Helath Reader. Vol. 1: Income Inequality and Health. New York: The New Press; 1999.
11. Marmot MM, Wilkinson RG, editors. Social Determinants of Health. New York: Oxford University Press; 1999.
12. Kawachi I, Berkman LF, Neighbourhoods and Health. New York: Oxford University Press; 2003.
13. Mackenbach J, Bakker M. Reducing Inequalities in Health: A European Perspective. London: Routledge; 2002.
14. Leon D, Walt G. Poverty Inequality and Health: An International Perspective. New York: Oxford University Press; 2001.
15. Kawachi I, Kennedy BP. The Health of the Nations: Why Inequality is Harmful to Your Health. New York: The New Press; 2002.
16. Ståhl T, Wismar T, Ollila E, Lahtinen E,Leppo K. Health in All Policies, Prospects and Potentials. Helsinki: Ministry of Social Affairs and Health; 2006.
17. Kickbusch I. Tackling the political determinants of global health. BMJ. 2005;331:246–7.
18. Sakellarides C. Stewardship. In: Marinker M. Constructive Conversations About Health. Policy and Values. Oxford: Radcliffe Publishing, 2006. p. 76–90.
19. Boerma JT, Stansfield SK. Health statistics now: are we making the right investments? Lancet 2007;369:779–86.
20. Murray CJL. Towards good practice for health statistics: lessons from the Millennium Development Goal health indicators. Lancet 2007;369:862–73.
21. Walker N, Bryce J, Black RE. Interpreting health statistics for policymaking: the story behind the headlines. Lancet 2007;369:956–63.
22. AbouZahr C, Adjei S, Kanchanachitra C. From data to policy: good practices and cautionary tales. Lancet 2007;369:1039–46.
23. Health at a Glance 2007 – OECD Indicators. [Online] OECD; 13 Nov 2007 [cited 10th Jan 2008]. Available from: miranda.sourceoecd.org/vl = 2288030/cl = 13/nw = 1/rpsv/health2007/index.htm
24. Kramers PGN. The ECHI project. health indicators for the European Community. Eur J Public Health 2003;13(Suppl. 3):101–6.
25. Eurostat. Structural indicators. [Online] Eurostat; 2007 [cited 10th Jan 2008]. Available from: epp.eurostat.ec.europa.eu/portal/page?_pageid = 1133,47800773,1133_47802588&_dad = portal&_schema = PORTAL
26. Lundgren B. 2004. Indicators for Monitoring the New Swedish Public Health Policy. Stockholm, Sweden: Unit Public Health Policy Anal., Natl. Inst. Public Health.
27. National Centre for Health Statistics. Healthy People 2010. Leading Health Indicators at a Glance. [Online] National Centre for Health Statistics: 2007 [cited 10th Jan 2008]. Available from: www.cdc.gov/nchs/about/otheract/hpdata2010/2010indicators.htm
28. European Commission Public health. Health strategy. [Online] European Commission; 2007? [cited 14th Mar 2008]. Available from: ec.europa.eu/health/ph_overview/strategy/health_strategy_en.htm
29. Loue S. Community health advocacy. J Epidemiol Community Health. 2006;60:458–63.
30. Boarini R, Johansson A, Mira d'Ercole M. Alternative Measures of Well-Being. OECD Statistical Brief No. 11. Paris: Statistical Directorate of the OECD; 2006 May.
31. Diener E. Happiness Accounts for Policy Use. Keynote Speech in International Conference: Is Happiness Measurable and What do Those Measures Mean for Policy? Rome, 2–3 April 2007. University of Rome "Tor Vergata" Italy. OECD; 2007
32. Canoy M. Well-Being and Policy Making. Presentation in International Conference: Is Happiness Measurable and What do Those Measures Mean for Policy? Rome, 2–3 April 2007. University of Rome "Tor Vergata" Italy. OECD; 2007

33. Veenhoven R. Measures of Gross National Happiness. Presentation in International Conference: Is Happiness Measurable and What Do Those Measures Mean for Policy? Rome, 2–3 April 2007. University of Rome "Tor Vergata" Italy. OECD; 2007

34. WHO Commission on the Social Determinants of Health. A Conceptual Framework for Action on the Social Determinants of Health. [Online] CSDH; April 2007 Draft. [cited 15th Jan 2008]. Available from: www.who.int/social_determinants/resources/csdh_framework_action_05_07.pdf.

35. Nolte E, McKee M. Measuring the health of nations: updating an earlier analysis. Health Aff 2008; 27:58–71.

36. Raffle AE, Alden B, Quinn M, Babb PJ, Brett MT. Outcomes of screening to prevent cancer: analysis of cumulative incidence of cervical abnormality and modelling of cases and deaths prevented. BMJ. 2003;316:901–5.

37. Danzon M. The values of values. In: Marinker M, editor. Constructive Conversations About Health. Policy and Values. Oxon: Radcliffe Publishining Ltd; 2006. p. 17–29.

38. Society at a glance 2005 – OECD Social Indicators. [Online] OECD; 2006? [cited 14th Mar 2008]. Available from: www.oecd.org/document/24/0,3343,en_2825_497118_2671576_1_1_1_1,00.html

39. Bauer G, Davies JK, Pelikan J on behalf of the EUPHID theory working group and the EUPHID community. The EUPHID health development model for the classification of public health indicators. Health Promot Int. 2006;21:153–9.

40. Agren G. Sweden's new public health policy. National public health objectives for Sweden. Report 2003:58. Stockholm, Sweden; Swedish National Institute of Public Health; 2003.

41. UNDP: United Nations Development Programme. Technical note 1: Calculating the Human Development Indices. United Nations Development Report 2006 [Online] UNDP; 2006 [cited 5th Sept 2007]. Available from: hdr.undp.org/hdr2006/statistics/documents/technical_note_1.pdf

42. Cobb C, Halstead T, Rowe J. The Genuine Progress Indicator: Summary of Data and Methodology. San Francisco: Redefining Progress; 1995.

43. Diener E. A value based index for measuring national quality of life. Soc Indic Res 1995;36:107–27.

44. Save the Children. The State of the World's Mothers 2002: Mothers and Children in War and Conflict. A Save the Children Publication. Westport: Save the Children; 2002.

45. Emes J, Hahn T. Measuring Development: An Index of Human Progress. A Fraser Institute Occasional Paper. (No. 36) Vancouver: The Fraser Institute; 2001.

46. Estes, R. Table 1: The Index of Social Progress (ISP2000, WISP2000). [Online] University of Pennsylvania [cited 5 Sept 2007]. Available from: www.sp2.upenn.edu/~restes/WISP2000/Table%201%20Indicators.pdf

47. Prescott-Allen R. The Well-Being of Nations: A Country-by-Country Index of Quality of Life and the Environment. IDRC/Island Press; 2001.

48. Boelhouwer J, Stoop I. Measuring well-being in the Netherlands: the SCP index from 1974 to 1997. Soc Indic Res 1999;48(1):51–75.

49. EUSI: European System of Social Indicators. Calculation of Composite Index of Individual Living Conditions. European System of Social Indicators [Online] GESIS German Social Sciences Infrastructure Services, ZUMA. Page last updated 2007 July 20 [cited 5 Sept 2007]. Available from: www.gesis.org/EN/social_monitoring/social_indicators/Data/EUSI/pdf_files/Doku_Index_Constr.pdf

50. Miringoff M and Miringoff M. The Social Health of the Nation: How America is Really Doing. New York: Oxford University Press; 1999.

51. Atkinson Foundation. Canadian Index of Well-being: Measuring What Matters. CIW [Online] The Atkinson Charitable Foundation [cited 5 Sept 2007]. Available from: www.atkinsonfoundation.ca/ciw/CIW_Brief_March_2007_MEDIA.pdf

52. Miringoff ML, Opdycke S. America's Social Health. Putting Social Issues Back on the Public Agenda. New York: ME Sharpe; 2008.

53. Desjardins and T. Schuller, editors. Measuring the Effects of Education on Health and Civic Engagement: Proceedings of the Copenhagen Symposium. OECD Directorate of Education, Centre for Educational Research and Innovation. Paris: OECD; 2006

54. Huisman M, Kunst AE, Bopp M et al. Educational inequalities in cause-specific mortality in middle-aged and older men and women in eight western European populations. Lancet 2005;365:493–500.

55. Pensola T, Martikainen P. Life-course experiences and mortality by adult social class among young men. Soc Sci Med 2004;58:2149–70.

56. Steenland K, Henley J, Thun M. All-cause and cause-specific death rates by educational status for two million people in two American Cancer Society cohorts, 1959–1996. Am J Epidemiol 2002;156:11–21.

57. Kuh D, Ben-Shlomo Y, Lynch J, Hallqvist J, Power C. Life course epidemiology. J Epidemiol Community Health 2003;57:778–83.

58. Ezzati M, Lopez AD, Rodgers A, Hoorn SV, Murray CJL and the Comparative Risk Assessment Collaborating Group. Selected major risk factors and global and regional burden of disease. Lancet 2002;360:1347–60.

59. McDowell I, Spasoff RA, Kristjansson B. On the classification of population health measures. Am J Public Health. 2004;94:388–93.

60. WHO European Centre for Health Policy. Health Impact Assessment. Main concepts and suggested approach. Gothenburg Consensus paper, Dec 1999. Copenhagen; WHO Regional Office for Europe: 1999.

61. Mindell J, Ison E, Joffe M. A glossary for health impact assessment. J Epidemiol Community Health 2003;57:647–51.

62. European Observatory on Health Systems and Policies, Wismar M, Blau J, Ernst K, Figueras J, editors. The Effectiveness of Health Impact Assessment. Scope and Limitations of Supporting Decision-Making in Europe. Copenhagen: Regional Office for Europe, World Health Organization; 2007.

63. Wismar M, Blau J, Ernst K et al. Implementation and institutionalizing HIA in Europe. In: European Observatory on Health Systems and Policies. The Effectiveness of Health Impact Assessment. Scope and Limitations of Supporting Decision-Making in Europe. Copenhagen: Regional Office for Europe, World Health Organization; 2007. p. 57–78.

64. Veerman L, Bekker M, Mackenbach J. Health impact assessment and advocacy: a challenging combination. Soz Praventivmed 2006;51:151–2.

65. European Commission. WHITE PAPER. Together for Health: A Strategic Approach for the EU 2008–2013. Brussels: Commission of the European communities; 2007

66. Seymour JD, Yaroch AL, Serdula M, Blanck HM, Khan LK. Impact of nutrition environmental interventions on point-of-purchase behavior in adults: a review. Prev Med. 2004;39(Suppl. 2):S108–36.

67. Fewtrell L, Kaufmann R, Prüss-Üstün A. Lead: assessing the environmental burden of disease at national and local level. Geneva, World Health Organization, 2003 (WHO Environmental Burden of Disease Series, No. 2)

68. Cole BL, Fielding JE. Health impact assessment: a tool to help policy makers understand health beyond health care. Annu Rev Public Health. 2007;28:393–412.

69. Boyd DR, Genuis SJ. The environmental burden of disease in Canada: Respiratory disease, cardiovascular disease, cancer, and congenital affliction. Environ Res. 2008 Feb;106(2): 240–9. Epub 2007 Sep 29. PMID: 17904543 [PubMed – in process]

70. Mindell J, Joffe M. Predicted health impacts of urban air quality management. J Epidemiol Community Health. 2004;58:103–13.

71. Valent F, Little D, Bertollini R, Nemer LE, Barbone F, Tamburlini G. Burden of disease attributable to selected environmental factors and injury among children and adolescents in Europe. Lancet. 2004;363:2032–9.

72. Stafford M, Cummins S, Ellaway A, Sacker A, Wiggins RD, Macintyre S. Pathways to obesity: identifying local, modifiable determinants of physical activity and diet. Soc Sci Med. 2007;65:1882–97.

73. Frank LD, Saelens BE, Powell KE, Chapman JE.Stepping towards causation: do built environments or neighborhood and travel preferences explain physical activity, driving, and obesity? Soc Sci Med. 2007;65:1898–914.
74. Gauvin L, Riva M, Barnett T, Richard L, Craig CL, Spivock M, Laforest S, Laberge S, Fournel MC, Gagnon H, Gagné S. Association between neighborhood active living potential and walking. Am J Epidemiol. 2008 Jan 27; [Epub ahead of print] PMID: 18227097 [PubMed – as supplied by publisher]
75. Kelly CM, Schootman M, Baker EA, Barnidge EK, Lemes A. The association of sidewalk walkability and physical disorder with area-level race and poverty. J Epidemiol Community Health. 2007;61:978–83.
76. Murray CJL, Lauer JA, Hutubessy RCW et al. Effectiveness and costs of interventions to lower systolic blood pressure and cholesterol: a global and regional analysis on reduction of cardiovascular-disease risk. Lancet. 2003;361;717–25.
77. Asaria P, Chisholm D, Mathers C, Ezzati M, Beaglehole R. Chronic disease prevention:health effects and financial costs of strategies to reduce salt and control tobacco use. Lancet. 2007;370:2044–53.
78. Haby M, Vos T, Carter R et al. A new approach to assessing the health benefit from obesity interventions in children and adolescents. Int J Obesity 2006;30:1463–75.
79. Segal L, Daziel K. Economic evaluation of obesity interventions in children and adults. Int J Obesity 2007;31:1183–4.
80. McPherson K, Marsh T, Brown M. Foresight Tackling Obesities: Future Choices – Modelling Future Trends in Obesity and the Impact on Health (2nd ed.). UK: Department of Innovation Universities and Skills, Government Office for Science; 2007.
81. Lopez AD, Mathers CD, Ezzati M, Jamison DT, Murray CJ. Global and regional burden of disease and risk factors, 2001: systematic analysis of population health data. Lancet. 2006;367:1747–57.
82. Powles J, Day N. Interpreting the global burden of disease. Lancet. 2002;360:1342–3.
83. Roosli M, Künzli N, Braun-Fahrländer C, Egger M. Years of life lost attributable to air pollution in Switzerland: dynamic exposure-response model. Int J Epidemiol, 2005;34: 1029–35.
84. Bere E, Veierod M, Skare O, Klepp KI. Free school fruit – sustained effect three years later. Int J Behav Nutr Phys Act. 2007;4:5–11.
85. Rodgers A, Ezzati M, Vander Hoorn S et al. Distribution of major health risks: Findings from the global burden of disease study. PLOS Med. 2004;1(1. e27):44–55.
86. Künzli N, Perez L. The Public Health Benefits from Reducing Air Pollution in the Barcelona Metropolitan Area. Barcelona: Centre recerca en epidemiologia ambiental (CREAL) Publication. 2007.
87. Suhrcke M, McKee M, Sauto Arce R, Tsolova S, Mortensen J. The Contribution of Health to the Economy in the European Union. Luxembourg: Office for Official Publications of the European Communities; 2005.
88. Mills PR, Kessler RC, Cooper J, Sullivan S. Impact of a health promotion program on employee health risks and work productivity. Am J Health Promot. 2007;22:45–53.
89. Miller P, Murphy S. Demonstrating the economic value of investments in health at work: not just a measurement problem. Occup Med (London) 2006;56:3–5.
90. Madon T, Hofman KJ, Kupfer L, Glass RI. Implementation science. Science 2007;318:728–9
91. Cohn D. Jumping into political fray: academics and policy making. IRPP Policy Matters 2006;7(3):1–36.

Chapter 3
Financing for Health in All Policies

Isabelle Durand-Zaleski, Karine Chevreul, and Gregoire Jeanblanc

Abstract Innovative public health policies that promote health and support the objective of Health in All Policies require innovative approaches in the allocation of resources. This chapter does not advocate any particular system of resource procurement and spending but compares the existing systems and attempts to understand how we can undertake health promoting public policies that do not increase the existing inequities in our societies. This chapter is not about public finance but about the motivation of policy makers and civil servants in charge of public money to support the Health in All Policies approach.

Policy innovations required to achieve 'Health in All Policies' upset the traditional ways of bureaucracies and health professionals. They affect the distribution of health and monetary benefits to the population. There is evidence that investing in health yields a two- to threefold return on investment, but those who are required to invest may not be the direct beneficiaries of that investment. Investment in innovative health policies may require a budget reform to allocate resources by missions that cut across institutions (both state and social health insurance (SHI) administrative departments). This might prove more difficult in countries with Bismarckian systems (SHI) where the state administration is traditionally in charge of public health provided by salaried state professionals while the SHI is in charge of health care with fee-for-service professionals. Thus coordination is needed between the two administration departments and their payment mechanisms.

The historical belief that economic growth results in improved health in developed countries has been contradicted by evidence from North America. Increasing income is not enough when the variables of interest for population health are the distribution of income and the social and cultural environment. Should policies target health determinants (or risk factors) one by one with specific policies or population groups? If the latter route is chosen, should measures be tailored to the requirements of specific populations or be universal. Evidence of successful interventions point at the combination of universal and specific measures. Targeting health

I. Durand-Zaleski (✉)
Universite Paris 12,Faculte de Medecine,Creteil, F-94010, France
isabelle.durand-zaleski@hmn.aphp.fr

I. Kickbusch (ed.), *Policy Innovation for Health*,
DOI 10.1007/978-0-387-79876-9_3, © Springer Science+Business Media, LLC 2009

determinants individually is easier because the tools already exists (monetary incentives, for example) but has so far had limited success on population health. Universal measures benefit the entire population, not those who need it most, but because of this, they tend to gain wider support from the general public. Specific measures which address the demands of those most in need have better face validity, but receive weaker political support. Policy innovation required to implement Health in All Policies seems cut across existing beliefs and bureaucratic domains and integrate interventions from administrative departments both at the national and local level with interventions from private stakeholders. Political involvement at the highest level is necessary to give the initial momentum, but sustainability at the local level requires the participation of local stakeholders in the policy design in addition to recurrent sources of revenues.

Introduction

The question addressed in this chapter is the relationship between funding (i.e., resource procurement in a publicly financed health care system), financing, and innovative public health policies. By 'funding' we mean social health insurance, taxes, or other mechanisms that provide the financial resources for implementing sustainable public health policies. Public health in developed countries now covers a wide range of issues: from traditional health protection to a wide range of preventative programs such as the prevention of domestic accidents, violence and road traffic accidents, substance abuse, environmental risks, and in the promotion of healthier lifestyles. Modern public health policies do aim not only to improve general life expectancy or the health expectancy of the individual but also to improve equity, solidarity, patient autonomy, and distribution of health in the population. Increasingly, public health deals with determinants of health that affect the spheres of influence, decisions, and, consequently, the budgets of government departments other than the health department. Public health policies also require sustainable funding, changes in behavior, and information systems

The fact that health is affected by policies in sectors other than health care (education, agriculture, transport, the law) has been recognized, but is not discussed in detail here [1] There is a growing body of literature on the broad scope of policies that influence the health outcomes of the population, including economic, education, and social services policies. One key issue for advocates of population health and actions on the social determinants of health is to reach policy makers beyond the traditional boundaries of health and social services. 'There is increasing recognition in the health promotion and population health fields that the primary determinants of health lay outside the health care and behavioural risk arenas. Many of these factors involve public policy decisions made by governments that influence the distribution of income, degree of Social Security, and quality and availability of education, food, and housing, among others. These non-medical and non-lifestyle factors have come to be known as the social determinants of health' [2].

The segmented approach of policy making (in education, the economy, the environment, and industry) limits the policy capacity of public health professionals. In order to act efficiently upon health determinants, public health professionals need knowledge of the potential consequences of policies carried out beyond the health care sector, and a critical mass of trained and influential people.

The focus of this chapter is policies that are typically labelled 'public health'. After presenting the background for Bismarckian and Beveridgian health systems, we will examine what financing mechanisms are required to promote and sustain policy innovation in health. We address the following issues: why it is important to innovate in health policy financing; why it is difficult; and how it can work? We conclude with examples and perspectives, using as an illustration the 2004 French public health and health care financing reform laws.

Background

European health systems have traditionally been described in terms of Bismarckian and Beveridgian systems. In Beveridgian systems, the state controls health and health care budgets, while in Bismarckian countries, health care is provided by medical professionals funded by Social Security payments (Social Health Insurance, or SHI, which includes statutory insurance, for example, sickness funds, retirement funds, accidents funds, and family funds), which in turn receives funding from employers and employees based on total payroll. This distinction, however, is becoming less and less relevant as far as the SHI revenues are concerned because most Bismarckian systems have to rely on additional resources taken from general taxation. It may still be relevant as far as the provision of services is concerned. In Bismarckian systems, there are two separate administrations, the state administration, which is predominantly in charge of public health and disease prevention, and the SHI administration, which is responsible for the provision of health care. Professionals in charge of health promotion and prevention, therefore, often belong to different administrations, both at the national and local levels and are paid a salary (in a state administration) or by a fee for their services (in the SHI system). In practice the distinction is often futile because office-based physicians are also involved in general disease prevention and health promotion, albeit on an individual rather than population basis. Germany is an example of adaptation of a Bismarckian system to the requirements of both health promotion and fee-for-service payment. Beginning in 1989 elements of heath promotion and prevention have been included in the mandatory benefit catalog of the sickness fund. Services to be included in the catalog and provided by fee-for-service physicians are negotiated between the funds and physicians' associations. The need for additional resources was recognized in 1995 by the Advisory council for the concerted action in health care [3]. Policies that require both interventions on health determinants and provision of health care services need to mobilize and pool resources from both state and SHI administrations. Acting on several determinants of health requires cooperation between administrations and payers both at the local and national levels. Beveridgian systems do not experience the separation between payers for health care and payers for action on social determinants that are built into Bismarckian systems. Bismarckian systems increase the number of stakeholders (administrations) involved at the national and, more importantly, at the local level. Such divisions between the national and local levels can be found for example in France or in Germany where health related responsibilities and decision makings involve the federal-level, state-level, and health-related areas [3]. It must also be understood that the umbrella term 'Social Security' covers a variety of insurance schemes that to not provide the same benefits to their members. Depending on the professional branch to which they belong, individuals contribute different premiums and are eligible for different benefits (e.g., the self-employed do not have the same contribution level as people who are salaried, and do not receive the same reimbursement rate for the health services they use). Thus, Social Security in Bismarckian countries often means several administrations whose contributors may have conflicting interests (Table 1).

We suggest, however, that the division between Bismarckian and Beveridgian systems as far as national health policies (both public health and health care policies) are concerned is almost a thing of the past. Bismarckian countries need to find additional resources for the ever-increasing deficit of the statutory health insurance. Recent reforms in France have broadened the revenue collection by introducing a income-tax-based contribution (e.g., in France roughly 40% of the Social Security budget comes from general taxes and the role of the state in the governance of the utilization of the health budget has increased since the introduction of the Social Security Financial Act in 1997).

Table 1 Distribution of responsibilities for health promotion and health care in Bismarckian systems

	Health care	Social determinants
National	Social Security: Statutory health insurance/ Sickness fund (several schedules and benefits)	Ministry of Health, other ministries, e.g., education, justice, finance, environment, family, youth Social Security: other funds, e.g., family, retirement, accidents
Local = region, state health-related areas	Local branches of Social Security/sickness fund	Local administrations for each ministry Local branches of Social Security
Professionals providing the services	Fee for service	Salaried
Reporting and indicators	Ministry of health and Social Security (sickness fund)	Ministry of health and other ministries such as Ministry of internal affairs, Social security
Legislation	Ministry of social services, prime minister, ministry of finance	Ministries of health, environment, finance, education, internal affairs, transportation, agriculture equipment . . .

Because of the EU policy to consider all expenditures from all public administrations together [4], policy makers in Bismarckian systems have a strong incentive to ensure that a decrease in state expenditures will not be offset by an increase in Social Security expenditures. There is a difficult equation because a decrease in public spending for selected services will result increased use of health care, For example, insufficient home services may result in prolonged hospital stay or futile use of health care professionals when social workers would be best suited for the services needed. At the same time the aging of the population will result in an increase in Social Security expenditures. It is then necessary for the state not only to anticipate this increase but also to design policies that will decrease both public expenditures and health care expenditures. The cumulated deficit of public and Social Security expenditures is now the figure of interest which creates a strong incentive for policy makers in Bismarckian countries to consider the health effects of all public policies.

In France, the first time the state and Social Security budgets were debated and voted for simultaneously by the French Parliament was in 2007. The justifications were that there is little difference to citizens between taxes and social contributions and that the EU reporting regulations concerns the expenditures of all public administrations in total.

We will argue that innovations in financing, although they do not constitute a policy innovation by themselves are necessary to ensure that policy innovations take place and become sustainable. We will therefore contrast innovations in raising new funds for health care and the financial reforms required by public health policy innovations, for example, by merging existing budgets that belong to different administrations. The ability of a country to engage in financial innovations is influenced by its health/health care financing system and by the legitimacy of the payer to act on the determinants of health. In a commercial insurance system, those who pay for damage have a straightforward authority to build in incentives that reduce risk, for example, by offering reduced insurance premiums to home owners who install burglar alarms. This simple framework cannot be applied to health promotion and health care. Although the Social Security pays for the treatments of diseases related to unhealthy lifestyles, its administration is hardly considered legitimate to influence peoples' lives. There are several explanations for this lack of legitimacy. One is that contributions are not determined by level of risk but by income level; another is that the link between a risk factor and a disease is not as clear as that between burglary and a burglar alarm. A third explanation is respect for individual autonomy and the thin line between offering legitimate information about healthy lifestyles and authoritarian interference to try and alter individual behavior. For example, the Social Security scheme for self-employed people in France adopted an incentive system that fully reimbursed the dental treatment costs for pastry shop workers who complied with preventive dental care. This experiment, although successful with regard to reduced tooth decay, was neither continued nor extended to other groups within the general population. The payer did not have the right to reward and therefore create a difference between individuals who had made identical financial contributions. We do not think that the legitimacy problem is specific to Bismarckian systems. We do not think that the legitimacy problem is specific to Bismarckian systems. In Beveridgian systems the State's ability to make individuals pay for maintaining unhealthy lifestyles can be questioned on the grounds that such policies harm the most fragile populations and may equally conflict with their values.

While illustrations of the importance of acting on the determinants of health will be drawn from all types of systems, description of the difficulties and possible solutions can be illustrated in greater detail with an example from a Bismarckian system, that of France

Why It Is Important to Engage in New Ways to Finance Public Health Policy Innovations

One of the most pressing needs for public health policies in developed countries is to reduce the inequalities in access to good health and to address the issue of the social determinants of these inequalities [5]. It is not morally acceptable to accept that diminished health is the result of poverty via a number of determinants such as poor diet, substance abuse, inadequate housing, and so on. Evidence on the determinants of poor health status and reduced life expectancy (for example, in the European population) is disturbing: (1) the health gap between social groups has not decreased globally in the past 20 years despite periods of sustained economic growth; (2) the health gap begins early in life, as early as 6 years of age for obesity, dental health and vision disorders; (3) poor health has a significant relation with almost every possible marker of lower socioeconomic status: low education level, unemployment, poverty, homelessness, single parenthood, mental health, violence, and substance abuse [6]. In European countries, for example, smoking contributes a large share of socioeconomic inequalities in mortality [7]. In France, the 7-year gap in life expectancy between the lower and upper social classes is largely explained by the effect of alcohol and tobacco abuse (30%), accidents, and suicide (15% and 11%, respectively) [8].

The hypothesis of a multiple way causal relationship has good face validity and implies designing an overarching policy to address the global needs of population groups rather than target each social determinant with a specific policy and specific subsidies [9]. It implies designing a policy that addresses the needs of adolescents in deprived neighborhoods rather than combining one policy to reduce substance abuse, another to fight eating disorders and a third to tackle sexually transmitted diseases, for example. The approach to health promotion has historically been segmented by provider while it is likely that coordination would improve overall efficiency.

We Classify Public Health Policies That Attempt to Reduce Health Inequities by Target and Instruments

The historical approach to public health interventions on social determinants of health is based on the segmented concept of risk and behavior. this approach uses financial incentives (positive or negative) to influence an individuals' behavior toward for example seeking employment, finding a home or smoking. Each risk constitutes a target and the instrument used to change behavior is uniformly financial incentives either positive or negative. In such an approach, policy makers take the (liberal) view that money is the means to achieve health [9]. If cigarettes are more expensive than fruit and vegetables, proponents of this policy expect that individuals will smoke less and eat a healthier diet. If low-income households can claim tax deductions for interest on loans, they are more likely to become home owners. This approach which establishes a direct link between income and health is attractive to policy makers who favor economic growth but ignore the health effects of wealth distribution [10]. A counter illustration is provided by the trends in Russia in early 2000, which combine economic growth with a decrease in life expectancy. [11]. Policies that reduce public spending (allegedly to increase the disposable income for households) but increase the inequalities in income distribution result in harmful health effects [10].

A second approach analyzes what are the effective public health interventions and which of these interventions are at least as effective in lower socioeconomic groups as they are among higher [7]. This approach considers each risk with a view toward the specific requirements of a population group; for example, smoking-cessation programs that provide the same benefit to individuals of lower socioeconomic status as they do to individuals of higher socioeconomic status. It is consistent with the theoretical framework that first, there is a relationship between health and wealth, and second, that this relationship is affected by the social and cultural environment.[10] Financial incentives should not therefore be the only instruments used but need to be complemented by specific services tailored to the needs of the population groups concerned.

A third approach argues for all-encompassing interventions which do not separate such determinants as education, employment, housing, and health [9]. In terms of allocating resources to public policies, it may require using the healthy-equivalent income [12, 13]. This indicator substitutes to the traditional objective of an identical health for all with the objective of equal standards of living. In terms of policy it means creating a weighted measure of health and income and designing public policies that result in an equal healthy-equivalent income for all. This indicator uses the willingness to pay approach in addition to the more conventional tools of accounting. For example, poor health is valued by the loss of income it generates to which is added the social willingness to pay for avoiding this poor health. Using this innovative indicator increases the income value of poor health and therefore the return on investments in health. It must be noted that there is indeed a political demand for approaches that allow qualitative measures to complement traditional wealth and well-being indicators (cross reference to Ildefonso chapter 2 [14]).

A less dramatic innovation is to acknowledge the fact that individual choices are to a large extend the result of social origins (e.g., smoking is considered a symbol of freedom by certain groups). The consequences for the choice of public health policy instruments are important. If individual choices are socially determined, it implies that individual incentives (supplemental income or negative incentives) must be complemented by global measures. Theses measures include recognition of the social rights of groups such as the unemployed or disabled people and participation of their representatives to policy making [9]. This third approach is consistent with the view that we need to shift from a financing model to an investment model. By this we mean that improving the condition of younger children for example is a joint investment by the departments in charge of education, housing and health care. The economic relevance of an investment in health has been promoted by the EU [15] and by the World Health Organizaton at the 6th Global Conference on Health Promotion [16]. When compared with the cost of doing nothing, investments in health promotion are estimated to generate net savings up to three times the initial investment. We will argue that these investments require not only support of all departments concerned but also an integrated provision of services. It implies an agreement at the government level on both the targets an the instruments of health policies.

The Appropriate Policy Level Needs To Be Defined

Public Health policies that address health determinants typically cut across the boundaries of administrations or services (cross reference to Morton Warner's chapter 5). The process involves the institution responsible for budget allocation, (often an administration or SHI but also increasingly nongovernment organizations, or NGOs), the providers and the ultimate beneficiaries. Table 2 summarizes some elements of comparison between health policies that take a sectoral versus global approach of social health determinants. The consequences for policy financing and provision of benefits are presented.

A sectoral public policy could be, for example, a flu vaccination program for the elderly in France. Specific funds are earmarked by the department of Social Security and people over 65 receive a letter inviting them to visit their general practitioner

Table 2 Health policies that concern one aspect of individual health or one health determinant (sectoral) versus policies that concern several interdependent health determinants (global)

Health policies: Sectoral vs global approaches	
Sectoral	**Global**
• Earmarked funds, benefits can be tied to previous contribution	• Several funding sources
• 1 type of service	• case management : multi disciplinary and multi-professional
• 1 type of provider	• Several administrations
• 1 administration	• Emphasis on social responsibility
• 1 group of beneficiaries	• Assessed on long term global indicators
• Emphasis on individual responsibility and behaviour	

(GP) to receive the flu jab. In economic terms, the justification for the Social Security department is that the elderly present a high risk of developing respiratory complications and the investment in immunization is offset by the reduction in hospital costs. In that case, the payer for the prevention policy is also the beneficiary of the investment. In the case of people under 65 who are currently employed, the department of Social Security has no financial interest in offering immunization because these people are at low risk of developing serious respiratory complications that would result in hospital admission. The major financial burden is on the employer. A sick employee not only has reduced productivity but also can infect others in the workplace. Thus for people under 65, the flu jab is often provided by the employer. Such sectoral policies omit certain members of the population (e.g., the unemployed or people whose employers do not offer an immunization program).

An example of a global public policy can be found in the 2008 French finance law for Social Security department. The objective, 'to prevent exclusion of vulnerable persons,' will be funded through Social Security and state sources and involves the services of both health and non-health professionals. This example will be presented in greater detail below [17].

Past Policies Have Not Been Uniformly Successful in Reducing the Negative Impact of Social Determinants on Health

So far, innovation in financing has mostly consisted of creating individual financial incentives for providers and users of the health care delivery system, or in looking at wider social policies, [such as]supplemental income for single-parent families, unemployment benefits, and low-cost housing. These individual incentives have proven their usefulness but they have the drawback of creating ceiling effects and stigmatization [9]. True policy innovation implies a multisectoral perspective and consideration of costs and incentives beyond the boundaries of health care. Financial strategies and tools can be innovative but are not in themselves a policy innovation. We will therefore examine what constitutes innovations in public health policy financing and how they affect either the expenditure or the revenue side and their impact on health.

Innovations in payment policies (expenditures) have been designed and used to solve problems of quality of care or to contain health care expenditures by encouraging a 'virtuous' behavior that reduces consumption through individual (financial) incentives. The case studies of financial incentives in European countries include Health Maintenance Organizations (disease management) experiments, prospective payment system in hospitals, pay-for-performance for providers, increases in of out-of-pocket costs through franchise and co-payments for patients. Innovation in payment policies have often been prompted by the need to reduce misuse, under- or more frequently overuse of health care The paradox may be that those payment innovations have little effect on the overall health of the general population because they affect the frequent users of the health care system (10–15% of the population). Other authors have commented on the uncertain relationship between payment incentives and health outcomes and on how short lived the effects on expenditures usually are [18].

Innovations that increase the money flow into the health care system may affect the population at large (instead of only the sick population) through general taxation, payroll taxes, VAT, and product-specific taxes. Research on the health and well-being effects of income and its distribution is still controversial, there is however evidence that income transfer programs which reduce the incidence of low income families have a favorable effect on healthy child development providing they occur in an environment of policy support that does not result in stigmatization or exclusion of a social group [19]. As noted earlier, the important factor is the social and cultural environment created by the overall policy rather than money transfers in themselves [10].

Policies that increase the costs to patients have been in the past combined with tax cuts in a general taxation package. This fiscal policy package was expected to render increases in patients' costs more acceptable to the voters. For example, in France the 2007 franchise on doctor's visits and the reduction in income tax were combined in the presidential fiscal policy package. Because such policies may harm the most vulnerable populations (sick persons) while benefiting taxpaying households (middle and upper classes), they ought to be combined with financial safety nets to preserve welfare benefits. They are otherwise likely to undermine the living conditions of underserved populations once by weakening public services and twice by increasing out of pocket costs [10, 20].

This brief overview underlines how much the approach to health problems has been segmented between prevention and care, provision of health care and social services, and the limited attempts at policy integration. There has been a tendency to increase segmentation rather than create one-stop shops where a full range of integrated services could be accessed without prohibitive time costs and cumbersome paperwork. Complexity increases when attribution of services in cash or in kind follows different rules, within one country: needs based, means tested, or conditional to previous contribution from the beneficiary. This complexity not only increases administrative costs but deters potential beneficiaries from seeking help and creates a rigid system which is not suited to the way family situations rapidly evolve nowadays. The option of an integrated and comprehensive policy appears to be the appropriate response to tackling interdependent health determinants [9]. This policy requires, at least in Bismarckian countries, a reform of the laws governing health care services [21] to allow better coordination and consistency in public health policies.

Why Is It Difficult to Finance Innovative Public Health Policies

Policy makers, however, experience difficulties in promoting the innovative financial policies needed for the implementation of innovative public health policies. There is a tendency to repeat or marginally change the same policies, because first there is too much to do and not enough policy support from the highest government levels and second bureaucracies and various interest groups join forces to oppose innovations that upset habits or rents.

There Is Too Much To Do and Not Enough Policy Support from the Highest Government Levels

Faced with the task of looking at what changes in the health determinants are required to achieve population health, policy makers may be tempted to give up. They argue that there is too much to deal with and they do not know where to begin. Researchers have evidence that the lifestyle (alcohol, tobacco, and fat consumption) the education, the neighborhood, the housing environment, the employment status, the working conditions and the financial situation are all statistically significant in relation to health and that poverty makes it even more difficult and costly to undertake health promotion actions [22]. In addition to having limited operational use, some of this evidence is not 'politically correct' (e.g., persons of lower socioeconomic status do not quit smoking as persons with higher socioeconomic status do)

As noted by Evans and Stoddart [10], the evidence on where to invest the money in order to achieve health benefits through health promotion exists but may not be presented and supported by a strong body of advocates. Interventions on health determinants also require coordination among advocates/stakeholders who have historically been engaged in providing support to different social or ethnic groups or doing research on one specific determinant, for example, tobacco consumption. These advocates belong to different worlds in the academia or NGOs and do not usually constitute a strong group of 'global population health' professionals. Their ability to divert resources from health care to health promotion has been limited. A more disturbing hypothesis is that policy makers at the highest level have privileged relationships with physicians and other health care professionals who are forceful advocates of health care spending, and fewer relationships with advocates of population health [23].

Although past investments in health care have historically had limited success in significantly reducing health inequities, policy makers are tempted to pursue them because of path dependency [24]. In developed countries departments have been put in place to distribute fund for specific interventions each one in their specific field (e.g., unemployment, housing, handicap, health care or public health, and so on). The theory of path dependency predicts that most policy changes will be incremental and will channel additional resources through the existing bureaucracies. In other words, path dependency implies that additional funds are more easily provided to existing programs than to new programs designed to respond to new demands. The current innovation in the French finance law for both state and Social Security budgets tends to contradict the theory of path dependency does not always occur; it is, however, too early to assess the effectiveness of both the anti discrimination and the active solidarity policies.

The Joint Interests of Bureaucracies and Various Interest Groups Oppose Innovations That Upset Habits or Rents

T. Oliver [25] proposed the following typology which is useful not only to explain past successes or failures of health policies but also to plan sustainable financing for future actions. Health policies are characterized by their benefits and sources of funding (Table 3).

Public health policies may benefit a large number of individuals who do not belong to identified interest groups or who do not feel related to one another by common interests. In that case the benefits of a policy will be considered 'diffuse'. By contrast, some policies specifically address either the requirements of an identified group (unemployed or disabled people) or an issue (lead poisoning or substance abuse). The beneficiaries from these policies will be a limited number of individuals. Symmetrically, the costs of a policy can be borne by a large population (e.g., additional taxes) or by a smaller group (e.g., price incentives for tobacco control).

Although this framework was developed for policy analysis in the context of the USA, it translates easily to the situation of welfare state countries, either Bismarckian or Beveridgian. Policies with concentrated costs and benefits (*interest group politics*) in welfare state countries are the traditional domain of private not-for-profit organizations (nongovernmental organizations, or NGOs) which receive and distribute resources to a limited number of identified stakeholders. These organizations undertake the public health policies that fall within their domains only and have to work in association with other partners in order to broaden the scope of the health policy. An illustration can be found in the policy for the prevention and treatment of HIV infection which combined state budgets with budgets from NGOs. Smoking cessation campaigns and support for the implementation of anti smoking regulation

Table 3 Framework for the political and financial analysis of health policies

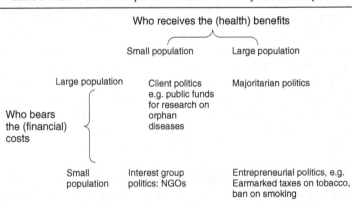

		Who receives the (health) benefits	
		Small population	Large population
Who bears the (financial) costs	Large population	Client politics e.g. public funds for research on orphan diseases	Majoritarian politics
	Small population	Interest group politics: NGOs	Entrepreneurial politics, e.g. Earmarked taxes on tobacco, ban on smoking

Table 3 adapted from Oliver [25]

are also often undertaken and financed by cancer support associations. In France, 'responsible contracts' involve private for profit or not for profit supplemental insurance companies who agree not to reimburse the co-payment due by patients follow the gatekeeping system and offer in their contracts measures of health promotions (e.g., promotion of health foods of healthy behaviors). Insurers may then claim tax deductions from the fiscal administration.

Such actions tend by nature to be limited in scope, however important within their domain. A policy addressing broader needs would require adding other resources to the support from NGOs.

By contrast, Oliver considers that a strong political commitment is necessary to obtain budgets for policies with diffuse benefits and concentrated costs (*entrepreneurial politics*) because of strong opposition from those bearing the costs or administrative bodies responsible for the budgets and weak support from the beneficiaries. This may not be so clear in welfare state countries which have traditionally used fiscal policy tools to increase the burden on least popular groups (e.g., smokers, alcohol drinkers, 4 Wheel Drive Vehicles (4WD) owners) in order to redistribute benefits to a larger population. The policy of increasing taxes on tobacco in order to reduce both active and passive smoking illustrates this policy as well as the tax on CO_2 emissions. An illustrative example is the smoking cessation policy in France. The price increase on tobacco (the earmarked tax created in the early 2000s) had an initial effect on cigarette sales which subsequently remained stable through the 2006–2007 ban on smoking which applied to the workplace and public places (with the exclusion of coffee shops, hotels, restaurant and discotheques). Enforcing the ban to all public places in 2008 apparently resulted in a dramatic decrease in acute vascular events as observed previously in Italy and the UK. In 2008 fear that the French government yield to the claims of tobacconists and coffee shop owners (those who allegedly bear the financial burden of the policy) prompted the French public health association to circulation a motion to support a total smoking ban [26].

Financing policies that benefit a small number of persons through measures that impose a small cost on a large population (*client politics*) is the usual method for health policies in welfare state countries. This is the preferred method for extending benefits to new population groups, for example, means-tested full medical coverage financed by general taxation, additional services for dependency and old age financed by a day worked but not paid for (Monday following Whit Sunday in France), and research institutions on specific topics (AIDS, orphan diseases) financed by general taxation and payroll taxes

Majoritarian politics where both payers and beneficiaries are numerous creates a possible case, even in welfare state countries, for involving multiple stakeholders both public and private at all administrative levels. In order to obtain a broader support for health policies, it might be interesting to move from client politics to majoritarian politics by demonstrating that the apparent benefit to a small number of persons affects in reality a much larger population. National campaigns to reduce obesity, for example, can benefit non-obese persons who will find greater availability of healthier foods or healthier means of transportation, or literacy programs also benefit literate persons by providing a more qualified labor force. A program of reduction of alcohol abuse may be supported by nondrinkers who expect a safer environment. The middle classes favor policies that benefit them (too) over policies that benefit only the lower-income groups. It is paradoxically a reason why universal (non means-tested) measures are preferred by policy makers. They gain wider support, better chance of being implemented and ultimately benefit the intended recipients. By contrast, means-tested measures may look more equitable but eventually never get implemented because of the opposition from non beneficiaries.

Financing Health Policy Innovation Requires Changes in the Process of Resource Allocation

Innovative public health policies require innovative financing. This means securing budget for the planned policy, defining payment mechanisms for providers and financial incentives for the population. The tools used for controlling health expenditures (negative financial incentives) have to be reversed to promote healthy behaviors or consumption. Tax deductions for healthy products only affect tax paying households. They could be combined with price deductions for tax-exempt households. Reimbursement of smoking cessation products and programs is already possible in some countries (usually with a ceiling). These approaches still consider health determinants separately; the single-problem approach, however, is now challenged in many countries.

The fact that public health policies create specific requirements with regards to income and income distribution has not yet been systematically recognized by public health laws enacted: as noted by Elbaum, only two out of the 104 priorities in the French public health law concerned health inequities [9]. Acting simultaneously upon several determinants of health requires cooperation between administrations and payers both at the local and national levels. Financing public health policies that deal with health determinants needs to cut across sectors (versus being directed to the health care sector). Beveridgian systems do not experience the separation between payers for health care and payers for population health that are built in Bismarckian systems. Bismarckian systems increase the number of stakeholders (administrative departments) involved at the national and, more importantly at the local level. What may appear as a drawback of Bismarckian systems may, however, prove an unexpected political advantage. Due to the separation of health care and health promotion budgets, health care professionals may not identify increases in budgets for health promotions as a threat to budgets for health care [10]. From experiments in both Bismarckian and Beveridgian systems the local level appears to be the appropriate one for implementing cross sectoral collaborations (cross reference to Morton's and Constantino's chapters 5 and 6). Difficulties to pool budgets or integrate services provided by departments that fight for budgets and territories are to be expected and need to be overcome by strong political leadership [27].

Financing for Innovative Health Policies

Role of the Health/Health Care Financing Model: Bismarck or Beveridge

In most European countries the State has a predominant role in ensuring health care and global population health. Systems in Europe have been described as 'social democratic', 'conservative', or 'liberal' This typology complements the more frequently used Bismarckian/Beveridgian distinction [20] for an analysis of the differences observed between European health policies. Bismarckian Social Health Insurance countries that tend to direct funds predominantly to health care must create new mechanisms to pay for public health at large and to finance sustainable way intersectoral actions. Countries with tax-financed health care systems have a tradition of setting apart budgets for intersectoral health promotion that far surpasses that of SHI systems. It may be due in part to the higher visibility of these budgets which are itemized whereas in SHI systems the health promotion actions performed by providers are not [20]. The most favorable setting for innovative health policies appears to be a Beveridgian system with a social democratic government. In such countries, state budgets can be allocated across sectors and the government ideology support generous public policies. In Bismarckian systems public policies can be generous if led by social democratic governments but the Bismarckian environment historically set limits to their scope. The limited past successes of collective health interventions in social health insurance systems have been noted and attributed in part to the focus on health care (rather than on population health) and in part to the lack of coordination between stakeholders [28]. Bismarckian systems deal with the purchase of primary health care to corporatist private providers whose fee schedule favors interventional individual care over population health. It might be a reason why the recent innovations were found in the publicly regulated hospital sector [28] rather then in the primary care sector. The increasing funding of SHI systems through taxes and private insurance might increase their ability to be involved in health promotion by making them more accountable to the general population [9]. A political act for SHI countries is to identify specific budgets directed to specific actors or institutions for cross-sectoral actions on the determinants of health. An example in France is the mode of financing the national health and nutrition program which concerned education (schools), city planning, health care, and health in the workplace. Another example is the recent national fund for solidarity and autonomy in France which integrates health care and social services at the national and local levels. Although these services are designed for sick patients, they create a framework that can be used more broadly. The national fund for solidarity and autonomy in France [29] is a one-stop shop for all benefits in relation to reduced autonomy. The provision is based on needs assessment with a list of the services required to maintain a persons' standard of living (e.g., housekeeping, home alterations, and medical supplies). The actual benefit is in cash, means-tested and paid only if the service is used.

Interventions on health determinants which break away from traditional policies and path dependency need secure recurrent financial resources. This is all the more difficult because innovative policies by definition have not been implemented before and therefore do not benefit from established budgets. Budgets for an innovation are voted as part of the country's finance law which are voted yearly, while innovative policies often require long-term investments or recurrent funds. There is no evidence that either Bismarckian or Beveridgian systems provide a better environment for sustainable funding: in both systems state budgets can be shifted depending on ministerial priorities and neither guarantees sustainability. One major advantage of Bismarckian systems may be that budgets are not tied to the election's calendar. When state budgets and Social Security budgets are pooled in the voting process this advantage may disappear. It is worth noting that this risk was somehow anticipated by the French public health law of 2004 law which established a secure 3–4-year budget. There might be discussion however as whether this time period is sufficient. Such was the case with health action zones [30]. 'An additional element of uncertainty for HAZs revolved around the issue of future funding. Although the zones had originally been launched with the promise of a 7-year life span, funding was never guaranteed. The initial budgets announced were only for 3 years and resources were allocated to HAZs on a yearly basis. The shift in ministerial priorities created considerable concern among project managers that the profile of the initiative at a national level had been diminished and that the future was more uncertain.'

The Geographical Level: National (Federal) or Local

Policy changes in either Beveridgian or Bismarckian countries pose the question of the appropriate geographical level of bureaucratic involvement. There is an agreement that more responsibilities must be given at local levels and that partnerships must be created between central & local government and health care providers, either the sickness funds or the National Health Service. Cross-sectoral policy changes are legitimate and sustainable when national and local policy makers have the ability to contract and pay providers, or remove financial disincentives [31]. The UK cross-cutting initiative illustrates how a cross-governmental strategy for tackling the causes of health inequalities operates at all levels [32] 'The theme is one of partnership, across Government and between Government and local communities'. These partnerships are not exclusively between public services but also involve voluntary groups (NGOs) and businesses or health care providers in private practice. Successful interventions in both countries are those that allow 'Re-orientation of resource allocation to enable systematic investment in community-based programs'.

If sustainable funding for one objective that requires the mobilization of resources from multiple bureaucracies is to be secured, evidence from France and the UK suggest that the highest level of political involvement, i.e. the prime minister and the Treasury is a success factor. Another recommendation is that 'policy formulation and implementation are interdependent activities,' which means that all stakeholders (all bureaucracies who will contribute to financing the policy innovation) are involved in the design of the policy and at the initiation of the process. This is often done in a perfunctory way by initially inviting representatives of the central administrations concerned. These representatives have the administrative legitimacy but lack the local legitimacy and convey a top–down management style ill-suited to the needs of local implementation. Designing the actions at the local level with a partnership between local representatives of the treasury and the other administrations involved, together with the voluntary groups and health care providers potentially concerned is recommended [33].

Before such dramatic changes in the balance of powers and the distribution of resources are implemented, consideration should be given to the stakeholders and their rationalities.

The Stakeholders and Their Rationality: What Are the Facilitating Factors for Successful Financing of Policy Innovation

Following the typology of Goddard et al. [27], we will examine how of politics, interest groups, bureaucracies and rent seeking stakeholders can facilitate or hinder the implementation of health policy innovations.

Politics and Majority Voting Models

Health policies, unlike health care reforms which concern mostly the limited number of sickness services, affect the entire population of a country or a region. Health (instead of health care) financing appears then a good opportunity for obtaining the support of voters who are concerned by health even if they are not usually concerned by health care. As noted by Kickbuch [34], national or local governments for SHI countries have had traditionally limited involvement in health care financing policies but are now becoming involved in financing health products and services beyond the traditional limits of health care. This occurs in Germany in the Berlin-Brandenburg region which has public support for health care, insurance, and health industries. In France, the government-supported plan to improve the quality of life of persons suffering from chronic diseases combines health promotion with provision of health care services [35]. The majority voting model would predict a rather good political support of budgets for health policies as every citizen may expect to benefit directly or indirectly from it. This may happen even when the government does not have the budget (in SHI countries) but is able to negotiate with the SIH the use of the budgets or to impose through legislation as in France and Germany/North Rhine Westphalia [36] to identify specific resources for the achievement of such health targets as ensuring equal access to care. Screening policies and the free prevention GP visit for every person aged 70 and over are examples of programs that are expected to benefit from a strong political support from vote-maximizing politicians.

Shifting away from health care and sickness services the unlimited demand for health reduces the pressure on health care expenditures. Access to health care until recently has not been constrained in Bismarckian countries with the result that health care services were occasionally used by consumers as health enhancement services. The need to contain public expenditures prompted reforms which limit both the access to health care providers and the quantity and quality of health care services provided. As health care becomes more constrained it may be anticipated that consumers will look into the market for health enhancement products (cross reference to Klaus chapter 4). This implies, however, that equity of access to those goods and services that affect health is ensured. Consumers need information and 'road maps' to navigate the second health market. It means at some point that positive discrimination in favor of those who need health literacy most can take place.

Budgets for targeted health policies may receive less public support. The option of financing those through the market or private insurance would result in the exclusion of the poorest. We suggest that health policies financed by public budgets combine high profile actions directed to the general population with population-specific community programs. This can be seen in the city of Nancy, which is part of the healthy cities program [37] and has implemented programs for the elderly and people in poverty which also benefit the rest of the population.

Health promotion may be a sound investment, but not necessarily for the stakeholder who actually made the investment. There are barriers to entry for policy innovations under the form of high sunk costs (irretrievable resources used in an education program, housing improvement, and so on) or high political risk. In that case policy makers are reluctant to commit resources unless additional information is provided to reduce the uncertainly [38]. This might be an important role for lobbies and interest groups who provide information to policy makers (cross reference to Ildefonso's chapter 2).

Interest Groups

Interest groups, private, and NGOs are frequently involved in the implementation and financing of health policies.

Interest groups and NGOs will favor policies as a rule that direct the benefits to their members while spreading the costs over the larger population [25]. The private sector is concerned with moral hazard and favors consumer incentives [39] to promote healthier lifestyle. Such actions were taken, for example, by a French private insurance company through discounts to enrolees purchases of health foods (this move was later on considered inappropriate and withdrawn by the company). NGOs financed health policies that are consistent with their overall objectives. An example can be seen in the health promoting hospitals initiative [40]. Thus the traditional care sector financed by sickness funds budgets and not state budgets can contribute to innovative health policy actions. Actions were financed by the hospitals' own budgets and addressed the health needs of their employees, patients and community As predicted by the interest group model, the budget was mobilized more effectively toward the hospitals' traditional customers. The programs most successfully developed through this initiative targeted patients and hospital staff, while actions in the community could be impeded by the legal difficulties and reluctance to use hospital budgets outside hospitals.

In a related way, employers are ready to participate to worksite health promotion projects that help improve employee morale and reduce direct and indirect costs of health failure, while employees would favor employer-provided paid time off during the workday and vending machine with healthier foods [41–43].

A majority of Fortune 500 companies undertake health promotion activities in the workplace. Among the factors identified as increasing participation rate, sharing (between employers and employees) costs, and time to participate in program activities appeared to play an important role [43] As each interest group tends to direct resources to the use that benefits itself most, some degree of coordination, tax incentives, and central planning is necessary to avoid imbalance in beneficiaries.

Bureaucraties

Bureaucracies tend to secure and expand their own budgets and favor policies that give them sole ownership of their funds. This, however, is contradictory with the needs of health policies. Budgets need to be attributed by missions/programs/actions which concern several ministries. Health promotion in the Netherlands faced 'a number of barriers which impede integrated policy development at the local level: the importance given to local health policy, the medical approach to health development, the organizational self-interest rather than public health concern, and the absence of policy entrepreneurial activity' [44]. Another experience was reported by the Canadian heart initiative which surveyed stakeholders of local health promotion policies: 'Respondents spoke often of barriers to integrated provincial chronic disease policy and action. The most commonly identified barrier was lack of financial resources and commitment by provincial governments for Chronic Disease Prevention and healthy living promotion strategies. This lack of funding and commitment was perceived to be related to competing priorities for policy attention and resource investment in acute care systems — areas considered to be in crisis by many provinces' [45]. A similar analysis was carried out in the UK, where the difficulties of implementing public health policies that tackle health inequities was traced to 'ministerial ambition, departmental survival, rigid boundaries, and inflexibility in public expenditure' The latter part is also described as a 'silo organization' in which public expenditures are authorized centrally and funds are allocated to each ministerial department [46]. Such allocation of resources contradicts the need for pooled budgets and cross-cutting initiatives. The health action zones initiative in England after the 1997 election illustrates some difficulties of Beveridgian systems to deal with pooled budgets and cooperation between administrations. Innovative public health policies still have to obtain earmarked budgets that come from different administrations and to use them consistently for a common goal. This program pooled funds totalling £152 million 'from several sources such as £21 m innovations fund, £90 m deprivation uplift and £30 m smoking cessation funding' [47].

Rent Seeking

In fee-for-service or capitation environments, health professionals have financial disincentives to engage in health promotion. These are expressed as lack of time and lack of training both of which can be translated into lack of specific compensation by the purchaser (sickness fund or community) [33].

Focus from both health care providers and the public is still on acute care and hospital care. The public is more concerned by the threat to local hospitals than by the lack of health improvement programs. An explanation might be found in the belief that each person is at risk for an acute event and might personally benefit from the money spent to keeping a hospital in operation whereas the benefits of public health interventions are diluted among a mass of unknown beneficiaries and individuals do not perceive the need for these services. This is a typical case for entrepreneurial politics where a policy maker with no fear of approaching elections is needed to show that there might be a statistical if not visible benefit of an intervention.

Opposition from health care providers is explained by the current payment mechanisms for physicians in primary care but also to a certain extent to that fact that specialists in public health retain their prerogatives. Thus, both groups appear to benefit from the current situation (or fear to loose from a different organization) and resist change. The reluctance from primary care physicians can be overcome by providing adequate training and removing financial disincentives. The resistance from office-based nurses may be both financial (as they are, like doctors fee for service) and cultural in countries where the tradition was for the nurse to 'work' for doctors and not for the community.

Case Study

Examples from the French Public Health and Health Care Financing Reform Laws

The French health care system belongs to the Bismarckian type and is typically not favorable to the population-based approach of health. The French laws on Public Health and reform of SIH, both voted within a few days in august 2004 demonstrate the disconnection between priority setting for public health and financing and also between bureaucracies in charge of each sector. The health targets selected in the public health law did not constitute a binding obligation for the SHI while the SHI law did not particularity address the issue of facilitating health promotion within the health care system.

Three years later however, the crisis in SHI finance prompted the system to reorganize the inputs and to seek new inputs, to use new modes of production and to develop innovative partnerships for financing and implementing policies. It is worth noting that the changes are still professionals centered rather than patient centered. The measures proposed for health promotion are few and, with the notable exception of weight control, not undertaken by health care professionals. The fact that objectives are spelled out in the Social Security finance laws means that resources are identified and earmarked to fulfil these objectives.

Finance laws for both the State budget and the Social Security budgets are subjected to the rules spelled out in 'organic' laws (laws on the law). Organic laws in 2004–2005 dramatically changed the paths of resource allocation for both budgets. They ruled that budgets will follow policy missions cutting across traditional administrative boundaries.

Solidarity and integration or health threats appeared as a state mission with a dedicated budget which cut across ministries and administrations. The state budget has 34 missions which may concern one or several administrations, such as solidarity and integration (several administrations), health (one administration), health safety (several administrations), social benefits, and pensions (several administrations). Departments responsible for each mission are required to define objectives and measurable indicators. An example of pooled state budgets is provided in the Loire region. The mission 'solidarity and integration' had a component of housing for homeless persons in winter time and a component of literacy. As winter was particularly mild the budgets for housing could be transferred to increase the literacy budget [48].

In 2007 the creation of the 'Haute Autorité de Lutte contre les Discriminations et pour l'Egalité' (HALDE or national authority to fight discrimination and enforce equality) and 'commissariat aux Solidarités actives contre la pauvreté' (commissioner in charge of active solidarity against poverty), both state institutions with missions to act upon health determinants might be a sign of change in the balance of advocacy powers and a shift from a sectoral to a global approach of health determinants The HALDE supports individuals or groups who are discriminated against when seeking employment, health care, housing, or in any other circumstance. It is also in charge of collecting and assessing interventions that reduce discrimination. The commissariat aux Solidarités actives contre la pauvreté' is in charge of fighting poverty through a number of interventions, such as the active solidarity income. The 'active solidarity income' is an experimental incentive designed to counteract the ceiling effects of the existing welfare benefits. In the current situation it might be more profitable for an unemployed individual to remain unemployed because an additional income would cancel eligibility to free supplemental health insurance, for example. The 'active solidarity income' combines the individual approach to financial incentives with overarching negotiations undertaken both at the local and national levels with employers, unions, and NGOs. These two institutions are expected to provide a global vision and additional policy support to the existing interest groups.

The 2007 organic law on Social Security ruled that each branch had to determine programs, objectives (targets) and indicators [49]. It created an obligation to set a budget for each program and to report on the spending and achievement of targets. This organic law has initiated a major shift from a spending to an investment model. The Social Security had historically been labelled a 'blind payer' which reimbursed providers without assessing the usefulness of interventions. The law made it an obligation to decide prospectively on the important issues in population health and to allocate resources accordingly.

For Health Care, the Programs and Targets Are [50]:

1. Ensure equal access to health care

   - Identify and reduce the percent of physician who bill over the official Social Security rate (e.g., 22 euro for a GP visit and 23 euros for a specialist visit) and reduce the average extra billing. In 2006, over 16% of the population lives in neighborhoods where over 50% physicians do extra billing and these physicians bill on average 50% over the official rate. This means that patients who have no or limited supplemental insurance have in effect reduced access to physicians in their neighborhood. The objective (not quantified) is to reduce both the number of physicians billing extra and the amount of extra billing.
   - Decrease the percent of patients eligible for state medical coverage who did not seek care for financial compared to patients with commercial supplemental coverage. In 2006 there was a 6% absolute difference.

2. Develop prevention

   - Reduce the percent of overweight and obese children (currently 15–20%), no targets
   - Reduce tobacco and alcohol consumption in the population over 15 years, from 25% of the population in 2007 to 24% in 2010 for tobacco and from 12.2 l in 2007 to 10.7 l of alcohol in 2010.
   - Increase breast cancer screening from 60% of the female population in 2007 to 65% in 2010 and cervical cancer screening from 65% to 80%
   - Increase immunization rate in children under 24 months from 88% to 95%
   - Improve oral health and decrease by 30% the rate of children with decayed teeth

3. Improve quality of care

   - Increase the current 85% rate of patients with a referring physician and the current 85% rate of primary visits to this referring physician
   - Improve coordination between hospital and ambulatory care by increasing over the current 85% the percent of territories where home care is available.
   - Increase from 93% to 100% the territories with 24-h emergency physician availability
   - Decrease waiting time for vital emergencies (no figure, the indicator has yet to be developed)

- Reduce to 0% from a current 2% the rate of hospitals that do not report hospital-acquired infections
- All physicians (100%) must undergo professional practice appraisal by 2010
- Increase the percent (from a current 11%) of health care organizations with the highest accreditation level

4. Improve efficiency and control health care expenditures

- Control the rate of increase of drug expenditures
- Increase over the current 75% the share of generic drugs (in number of boxes) sold
- Decrease the average number of drugs per prescription (currently 3) and the percent of prescriptions with six drugs or over (currently 10%)
- Decrease prescriptions for discharged patients
- Decrease the number of DDD per 1000 patients for antibiotics below the current 31 (highest level in Europe).
- Decrease the amount of compensation for leave of absence (currently 10% of all ambulatory care expenditures)
- For patients who are eligible for 100% coverage of health care expenditures in relation with a chronic condition, ensure that only expenditures in relation with that condition are fully reimbursed by the Social Security and that unrelated expenditures are reimbursed at the usual (65–80%) rate. It is expected that 75% of expenditures for patients with a chronic condition are related to that condition.
- Increase over 50% the rate of hospitals signing contractual agreements to limit expenditures on drugs and ambulance.
- Decrease prescriptions by office-based physicians (antibiotics, statins, proton-pump inhibitors, angiotensin-converting enzyme (ACE) inhibitors.)
- Increase to 85% in 2010 the proportion of ambulatory procedures for cataract surgery, knee arthroscopy, tonsillectomy, varicose veins, and teeth.
- Increase transfers and decrease waiting time from acute care to rehabilitation centers
- Increase hospital productivity

5. Ensure financial sustainability

- Reduce the current deficit
- Increase noncontribution revenues (fraud, abuse, unclaimed assets)

What can be deducted from these objectives and indicators is an endeavor to improve the fairness and efficiency of the system and financial sustainability without negative effects on health and health equity. The objectives are for 'patients' (consulting a physician with a health complaint) rather than the population at large, except in the case of prevention concerning obesity, tobacco, and alcohol consumption.

Safety in the Workplace

1. Reduce the incidence of accidents in the workplace, during transportation and prevent professional exposure to risk factors
2. Improve information on accidents and professional risks and ensure fair compensation
3. Ensure financial sustainability

Retirement Pensions

1. Ensure fair standards of living for retired persons
2. Increase choice for the age of retirement
3. Ensure solidarity between retirement benefits
4. Increase employment for elderly workers
5. Ensure financial sustainability

Family Benefits

1. Ensure fair compensation of family-related expenditures
2. Enable families to combine professional and family life
3. Support vulnerable populations: there are indicators relevant to health policy issues which are the number of children under age 18 who live in families below poverty threshold/unemployed with a current 8% figure and a 7% objective for 2010, the reduction of poverty with an objective of reducing the difference between the poverty threshold, and the actual average standard of living of households below poverty threshold from 16% in 2007 to 7% in 2010.
4. Ensure financial sustainability

Funding and Financing

1. Ensure fairness in financial contribution from households
2. Balance Social Security revenues with sustainable employment policies
3. Improve management
4. Ensure financial sustainability

Solidarity to Sustain Autonomy

1. Ensure fair standard of living for handicapped persons
2. Respond to the need for autonomy of handicapped persons
3. Respond to the need for autonomy of elderly persons
4. Ensure financial sustainability

These objectives can be compared to the 104 health targets spelled out by the 2004 public health law, but public health laws are not finance laws, which means that they do not necessarily tie resources to objectives, and public health targets *do not constitute a binding obligation for financing organizations* [50]. Baseline figures and trends for some of the 2004 health targets were clearly used to define specific objectives of the finance law, not only for health care programs but also for workplace safety and environmental safety. In addition to the indicators presented above, follow up on the 104 targets included air pollution, water pollution, and lead poisoning. Thus, health-related data were used to allocate state resources for missions outside the health care system (cross reference to Ildefonso chapter 2, [51]).

In addition to the State budget reform, the creation of an instrument labelled 'public interests partnerships' has allowed allocation of resources across administrative boundaries. This partnership is usually a short-lived contract with a specific policy objective. It is available to any department that needs to pool resources either with other departments at the national or local level or with a private partner. Public interest partnerships allow pooling of both public and private money for a definite objective and over a determined period of time. If the objective is more long term however, (e.g., international cooperation for health promotion) the partnership can have an undefined lifetime. In the field of health promotion a current partnership includes the national sickness fund, supplemental (private) insurance, and hospital federations, together with the Ministry of Health [52].

Conclusion: New Modes of Producing Health

The French example shows that the objective of improving population health can be incorporated in a Social Security finance law. The means to achieve the objective, however, are traditional rather than innovative. Finance laws plan for material inputs, which is not enough for the innovations in the organization of care. The proposed innovations consist mostly of using more efficiently the existing inputs or purchasing new inputs. One important structural aspect of SHI [28] is the fee-for-service payment based on the national agreements established between payers and health care professionals. Promoting prevention and education has required the adoption of a gatekeeping-like system with the gatekeeper being contracted for the management of patients' health. The gatekeeper or manager of patient health do not need to be a physician but this shift conflicts with corporatists interests and with the traditional culture of nurses and other health professionals who were traditionally 'commissioned (or prescribed)' by physicians and not by the community. Purchasing services for a population (instead of patients) does not come naturally to SHI systems mostly because those services were traditionally outside their missions (e.g., immunization, screening, and education). Contracting health care providers to produce health in addition to health care has been so far the preferred mode but new technologies render possible greater patient involvement. Patient involvement can be expected both in an active way as a coordinator of his own care and in a more passive way benefiting from a personalized health prevention through progress in genetic prediction.

G. Mulgan [53] suggests that innovation in health policies require social innovation which in turn has to be accompanied by a reorganization of administrations and changes in the boundaries and in the methods of coordination between administrations as well as between administration and NGOs. There is also a need to shift from the traditional view that promoting health means financing physical inputs. Producing health in the future will be producing knowledge that can be used by policy makers and patients (by opposition to the past situation of producing knowledge that was used predominantly by health professionals and academics).

Advocacy for population health requires knowledge brokers between public health academics and policy makers to highlight the policy implications of academic work (reference to Morton Warner's chapter). Promoters of innovative policies need to find common ground between groups that have no history of working together and may not share the same culture [54]. Symmetrically knowledge brokers have to assist professionals and patients (cross reference to Constantino Sakallides's chapter 6) in order to shift decisions regarding the management of individual health.

Health policies are satellites of public policies. A policy that addresses the broad determinants of health requires specific cross-sectoral and cross-ministries budgetary process and more broadly devolution of responsibilities to the local level or to the private (for profit or not for profit sectors). These financial requirements of health policies, although technical, may conflict with the government's ideology [19] when the government is leaning toward a 'liberal' (right wing) policy. Actions on health determinants take the view that social responsibility is predominant. Sustainability (economic, environmental and social) can cement administrations and NGOs that may take different view of individual and social responsibility but agree on the necessity to ensure that the population, the economy, and the territories where both operate will survive. These actions are more likely to be successful when undertaken at the local level where networks for health can be built into the workplace or in neighborhoods [36].

The historical belief that economic growth would result in improved health in developed countries has been contradicted by evidence from North America. Increasing income is not enough when the variables of interest for population health are the distribution of income and the social and cultural environment. Should policies target health determinants (or risk factors) one by one with tools or population groups? If the latter is chosen, should measures be tailored to the requirements of specific populations or be universal. Evidence on successful interventions points to the combination of universal with specific measures. Targeting health determinants individually is easier because the tools exists (monetary incentives, for example) but has had so far limited success on population health. Universal measures benefit the entire population, not those who need it most but because of that they gain a wider support. Specific measures have better face validity as they address the demands of those most in need but have weaker political support. The policy innovation required seems therefore to cut across existing beliefs and bureaucratic territories.

References

1. Health in All Policies, Edited by Ståhl T, Wismar M, Ollila E, Lahtinen., Leppo K Ministry of Social Affairs and Health, Ministry of Social Affairs and Health, Health Department Helsinki Finland 2006. Available at http://www.euro.who.int/document/ E89260.pdf?bcsi_scan_185FE7D7897B7B4A?0&bcsi_scan_filename?E89260.pdf

2. Raphael D, Bryant T. Researching income and income distribution as determinants of health in Canada: gaps between theoretical knowledge, research practice, and policy implementation. Health Policy 2005;72:217–232.

3. Public Health Policies in the European Union. Holland & Mossialos ed. Ashgate Publishing 1999 Aldershot, England.

4. http://www.performance-publique.gouv.fr/les-ressources-documentaires/les-publications-de-la-db/budget-infos-la-lettre-electronique-de-la-direction-du-budget/budget-infos-n1/dossier/ dossier-1-2.html

5. Whitehead M. Diffusion of ideas on social inequalities in health: a European perspective. Milbank Q 1998;76:469–492, 306.

6. Elbaum M. Social inequalities in health and public health: from research to policies Revue d'Épidémiologie et de Santé Publique 2007;55:47–54.

7. Kunst A.E. Describing socioeconomic inequalities in health in European countries: an overview of recent studies. Revue d'Épidémiologie et de Santé Publique 2007;55:3–11.

8. Programme de qualité et d'efficience maladie, LFSS 2008; p. 27. Available at http:// www.securite-sociale.fr/chiffres/lfss/lfss2008/2008_plfss_pqe/2008_plfss_pqe_maladie.htm

9. Elbaum M. Protection sociale et solidarité en France (Welfare and solidarity in France). Revue de l' l'Observatoire Français des Conjonctures économiques. 2007;102:659–622.

10. Evans RG, Stoddart GL. Consuming research, producing policy? Am J Public Health 2003 r;93:371–379.

11. World Bank WDI 2005; WHO/EURO HFA database 2005.

12. Fleurbaey M. Healthy-equivalent income, a tool to analyze social inequalities in health. Revue d'Épidémiologie et de Santé Publique 2007;55:39–46.

13. M. Fleurbaey et G. Gaulier, << International Comparisons of Living Standards by Equivalent Incomes >>, WP CEPII n° 3, janvier 2007; http://www.cepii.fr/anglaisgraph/workpap/ summaries/2007/wp07-03.htm

14. http://www.strategie.gouv.fr/IMG/pdf/NoteVeille91.pdf

15. Suhrcke M, McKee M, Arce RA, Tsovola S, Mortensen J. The Contribution of Health to the Economy in the European Union. European Commission, Health & Consumer Protection Directorate-General, Luxemburg Office for Official Publications of the European Communities, 23 August 2005.

16. http://www.hp-foundations.net/

17. Kesteman N. Évaluer les performances de la branche Famille. Des indicateurs prévus par la LOLFSS et la LOLF CNAF Recherches et Prévisions n° 88 – juin 2007.

18. Fielding JE, Lancry PJ. Lessons from France–'vive la difference'. The French Health Care System and US Health System Reform. JAMA 1993 11;270:748–756.

19. Raphael D, Macdonald J, Colman R, Labonte R, Hayward K, Torgerson R. Researching income and income distribution as determinants of health in Canada: gaps between theoretical knowledge, research practice, and policy implementation. Health Policy 2005;72: 217–232.

20. Raphael D, Bryant T. The state's role in promoting population health: public health concerns in Canada, USA, UK, and Sweden. Health Policy 2006 22;78:39–55.

21. Henke K-D. The funding and purchasing of healthcare. A book with seven seals. J Public Health 2006;14:385–390.

22. Linda I. Reutter, Gerry Veenstra, Miriam J. Stewart, Dennis Raphael, Rhonda Love, Edward Makwarimba, Susan McMurray Lay Understandings of the effects of poverty: a Canadian perspective Health & Social Care in the Community 2005;13: 514–530.

23. Lavis JN, Ross SE, Stoddart GL, Hohenadel JM, McLeod CB, Evans RG. Do Canadian civil servants care about the health of populations? Am J Public Health 2003;93:658–663.
24. Rochaix L, Wilsford D. State autonomy, policy paralysis: paradoxes of institution and culture in the French healthcare system. J Health Polit Policy Law 2005;3.0:97–119.
25. Oliver T. The politics of public health policy. Annu Rev Public Health 2006;27:195–233.
26. http://www.oft-asso.fr/pdf/Janvier%202008%20Indicateur%20mensuel%20ETS.pdf
27. Goddard M, Hauck K, Preker A, Smith PC. Priority setting in health — a political economy perspective. Health Economics, Policy and Law 2006;1:79–90.
28. Social Health Insurance systems in Western Europe, Saltman R, Busse R, Figueras J (eds). European observatory. Maidenhead, England: Open University Press; 2004.
29. http://www.sante.gouv.fr/htm/actu/31_050223.htm
30. Bauld L, Judge K, Barnes M, Benzevalm, Mackenzie M, Sullivan H. Promoting social change: the experience of health action zones in England. J Soc Policy 2005;34:427–445.
31. Rodwin VG, Le Pen C. Health care reform in France – the birth of state-led managed care. N Engl J Med 2004;351:2259–2262.
32. http://www.hm-treasury.gov.uk/media/B/8/Exec%20sum-Tackling%20Health.pdf   accessed August 2007.
33. http://www.renewal.net/Documents/RNET/Research/Tacklinghealthpractice.pdf
34. Kickbuch I. Innovation in health policy: responding to the health society. Gac Sanit 2007; 21:338–342.
35. http://www.sante.gouv.fr/htm/dossiers/plan_maladies_chroniques/plan.pdf
36. Health targets. Marinker M (ed.) BJM Books, London; 2002.
37. http://www.euro.who.int/healthy-cities accessed August 2007.
38. http://siteresources.worldbank.org/HEALTHNUTRITIONANDPOPULATION/Resources/28 1627-1095698140167/Chapter3Final.pdf
39. Janus K. Medicare as incubator for innovation in payment policy. J Health Polit Policy Law 2007;32(1):293–306.
40. http://www.euro.who.int/Document/IHB/hphseriesvol2.pdf accessed August 2007.
41. Linnan L, Weiner B, Graham A, Emmons K. Manager beliefs regarding worksite health promotion: findings from the Working Healthy Project 2. Am J Health Promot 2007;21:521–528.
42. Kruger J, Yore MM, Bauer DR, Kohl HW. Selected barriers and incentives for worksite health promotion services and policies. Am J Health Promot 2007;21:439–447.
43. Downey AM, Sharp DJ. Why do managers allocate resources to workplace health promotion programmes in countries with national health coverage? Health Promot Int 2007;22:102–111.
44. Hollander RB, Lengermann JJ. Corporate characteristics and worksite health promotion programs: survey findings from Fortune 500 companies. Soc Sci Med 1988;26:491–501.
45. Hoeijmakers M, De Leeuw E, Kenis P, De Vries NK. Local health policy development processes in the Netherlands: an expanded toolbox for health promotion. Health Promot Int 2007;22:112–121.
46. Robinson K, Farmer T, Elliott SJ, Eyles J. From heart health promotion to chronic disease prevention: contributions of the Canadian Heart Health Initiative. Prev Chronic Dis 2007;4:A29.
47. http://www.minefi.gouv.fr/lolf/downloads/710_annexes_r_16_09_05.pdf
48. http://www.finances.gouv.fr/lolf/4clics/clic4_01.htm
49. http://www.securite-sociale.fr/chiffres/lfss/lolfss/lolfss.htm
50. Durand-Zaleski I. Health targets in France: role of public health and social health insurance reform laws. Euro Health 2006;3:18–20.
51. http://www.sante.gouv.fr/drees/etude-resultat/er-pdf/er623.pdf
52. http://www.cnsa.fr
53. http://www.youngfoundation.org/node/274?bcsi_scan_F6BB184018017D9D = nWSafiy-ISAOo0y7 + 75h9/QgAAAA5R/EL
54. Cohn D. Jumping into the Political Fray: Academics and Policy-Making. May 2006 Vol. 7, No. 3. Institute for Research on Public Policy Matters, IRPP Montreal, Quebec.

Chapter 4
Health as a Driving Economic Force

Klaus-Dirk Henke and Karl Martin

Abstract This chapter illustrates the contribution which could be made to realizing the Lisbon Strategy of the European Union for growth and jobs by innovative health care policy favoring a preventive orientation of health care. The prevention and control of risk factors for chronic diseases, as well as their potential impact on the quality of human capital as a union of health and education, are discussed. Human capital refers to health and education both of the individual, and of the population as a whole.

Investments in health and education could be used to mitigate or compensate the negative consequences of demographic change and globalization. This chapter concentrates on how exhausting the prevention potential of chronic diseases could extend the labor force potential beyond the conventional age limit of 65 years. Labor force potential usually refers to the maximum supply of labor available from workers, the unemployed and other nonworkers within an age range of 20–65 years. This optional innovative policy is explained using the example of the development of labor force potential in Germany between 2002 and 2050, prerequisites being a change in health care policy from cure to prevention, as well as a cultural change. Cultural change in the population and in politics would mean attributing the same level of importance to the prevention and control of risk factors for chronic diseases as to the prevention and control of infectious diseases.

The accumulation of human capital through investments in health and education is crucial to the innovative competences of the population. Both these sectors promote growth in the remaining sectors of the economy and, through their own development, become an essential driving force of growth themselves.

The increasing demand for new products and services will create a second health care sector for health-related services combining services which are covered by the insurance and by private out-of-pocket expenditures. This second sector deals not only with care but also with goods and services aside from services covered by the insurance.

K.-D. Henke (✉)
Technische Universität Berlin, Fakultät VIII Wirtschaft und Management, Institut für Volkswirtschaftslehre und Wirtschaftsrecht

I. Kickbusch (ed.), *Policy Innovation for Health*,
DOI 10.1007/978-0-387-79876-9_4, © Springer Science+Business Media, LLC 2009

Expenditure on health and education therefore has to be included as an investment within the national accounts statistics, expanding upon the previous concept of investment. This in turn means that corresponding coefficients, for example, would have to be developed for health impact assessment purposes.

Expanding labor force potential via compression of morbidity and mortality requires that health and education policy be embedded in growth-orientated labor and economic policies in order to ensure that the potential working years gained have an impact on production and prosperity. Health in All Policies becomes imperative.

Starting Point: The Downsides of Cost Increases and the Upsides of Growth Effects with Regard to Health

In most countries health policy discussions revolve around cost containment. Both the Beveridge and the Bismarck systems focus on expenditure development. The OECD regularly records and compares *per capita* health expenditure with regard to gross national product, functions and the pharmaceuticals industry [1]. The social insurance systems additionally include contribution rates, both over time and separately for employers and employees.

Yet regardless of how the health care sector is documented and measured in monetary terms, whether based on expenditure or contribution rates, no ideal health quota exists. There is no practicable conclusion to be deduced using scientific means as to whether a state should spend more or less on nursing care, prevention, and health promotion. There are good arguments to spend more on prevention but at the same time nursing home care of the elderly needs more attention too. Bearing this in mind, it is imperative that we put a stop to the traditional argument that rising expenditure in health care leads to a cost explosion, that is, that a higher percentage of health care expenditure with regard to gross national product (GNP), or higher contribution rates, is necessarily a negative thing and that labor costs are fundamentally too high.

In all countries the health care allocation is taken from national economic resources, which are always marginal. Viewed globally, health care has to compete for these resources with climate protection measures, education, and research expenditure, the safeguarding of pensions, family policy and other areas besides. Expenditure in one area amounts to opportunity costs in another area.

From this macroeconomic viewpoint, the political decision-making process, coupled with market economic processes, leads explicitly or implicitly to the means or resources allocated to the health care sector within any one country.

Within the health care system there is then second-level competition for these resources between areas as diverse as prevention and health promotion, curative and emergency treatment, rehabilitation, nursing care, and palliative medicine, not to forget expenditure for statutory sick pay.

Focusing on individual patients, it is possible to categorize clinical diagnosis according to the International Code of Diseases and population groups e.g. by age and/or sex [2]. From this epidemiological perspective the goals of health care policy then become avoidable diseases and avoidable mortality. On this basis the burden of diseases can be demonstrated.

Finally, insured parties are interested in adequate insurance which in addition to basic cover also includes the option of extra individual care.

This observation of resource allocation has so far been functional, that is, independent of individual nations or time periods, but there is a more institutional view of the matter which also requires consideration. Within each country a comparison is made between the bodies occasioning expenditure, for example, the various branches of a national insurance system, private insurance or the individual budgets within health care systems financed by tax income.

The results of resource allocation generally attract too little notice, giving rise to a chiefly input-orientated view of the matter. This view is gradually becoming replaced by a desire for a more output-orientated view. With regard to the health care system, this means that the resources should be used where they "buy the most health". Ideally, expenditure would then have to be repeatedly restructured until the health benefits were equalized across the board. Or put another way: expenditure must be cut in those areas where wastefulness and inefficiency are greatest. Program and management-based efficiency increasingly have to replace the input orientation which still predominates [3].

Dissolving the input viewpoint based on expenditure or contribution rates throws up a need for result indicators. Such indicators are established and compared with the characteristics of different national health care systems in mind. Here the question arises of how these indicators are to be measured, and which ones are to be used for comparison purposes [4]. Upon which values and concepts is the selection based anyway: those of epidemiology, medicine, health economics or health policy?

In this context there has been a paradigmatic change, taking place in the different countries at different points in time and in some still ongoing. This refers not only to the aforementioned change away from the cost containment discussion and input viewpoint toward an output-orientated viewpoint, for example, avoiding diseases and death or increasing prevention and health promotion. We are primarily referring to the fact that health care is increasingly being acknowledged and classified in positive terms as a labor-intensive growth industry.

This perspective also requires that the selected indicators be substantiated, so that the effects of the health care sector on the national economy such as value added, employment and economic growth are operationalized. Here we are not just concerned with the markets for goods and services and the fiscal effects of health, health care and health systems, but also with the so-called factor markets; that is, in addition to the money and capital markets, these markets especially include the employment markets, with their manifold and new areas of occupation within the health care sector.

In Germany this discussion began with two reports by the Expert Council for Concerted Action in the Healthcare System in 1996/97 [5]. In the second volume the effects of health care on welfare, growth, productivity and employment were investigated for the first time and empirically assessed. In addition, progress in medicine and its various phases was addressed, evaluation and health technology assessment, as well as the role of university hospitals in the progress process and the financing of health-related research. Following an analysis of individual examples of medical progress and their respective economic viability, selected growth markets were then subjected to a broader exposition. Even back then this particularly included nursing care, medical telematics, medical products, and the pharmaceuticals industry with their individual growth potentials [6].

Ten years later, at least in Germany, the health care economy has not only become socially acceptable [7], but has also been addressed in its regionalism [8]. In 2008 the regional health care markets are also playing an increasingly significant role in the German government's research program.

Independently of the development in the industrial nations, the macroeconomic significance of health care investments can be seen within the context of economic development and globalization [9]. The EU is also seizing upon this context and is examining the contribution of health care to the national product of its member states [10].

Theoretical Considerations: Health as a Component of Human Capital

Discussion about the health economy as a growth industry now not only includes the abovementioned linking of health-related investments to growth, but additionally focuses on the foreseeable demographic development. Many experts neglect the potentials for growth and higher revenues in the face of increasing expectations within a population keen to enjoy healthy ageing. Yet healthy ageing as a growth determinant is a topic in itself.

Changes in the disease distribution, are partially linked to demographic developments. In particular, an increase in chronic diseases can be observed. Allergies, asthma, and diabetes are becoming widespread, due in part to ageing, and to environmental changes [11]. Thus, the medical treatment and disease management of patients with chronic diseases will increasingly substitute the treatment of acute diseases. From a population health view, the challenge of the future is the prevention and early diagnosis of chronic diseases.

Considering the changes in demographic development and morbidity structure of the population of highly developed countries, a gain in healthy and productive life years will be essential in order to maintain a high economic standard. Therefore, it will be necessary not only to improve the efficiency of health care delivery and financing instruments, but also to increase investments in health. As the former EU Commissioner David Byrne puts it: "Health Equals Wealth". This strong relationship led him to consider a health status indicator as a new, additional convergence criterion for the expanded European Union [12].

Given this background, two considerations justify the working hypothesis that there are growth and fiscal effects of better health [13]:

An improved health status is an investment in human capital, and alongside (private and public) capital and technical progress human capital is one of the three factors which explain economic growth and fiscal stability. A healthier population is more productive, and a higher functional capacity in an ageing population leads to economically productive life years. Improvements in health and education of the population are thus key factors in promoting growth and this also creates better quality of life for citizens.

On this basis new markets are opening up, not only in health care itself but also in other areas, such as wellness and fitness, nutrition, etc., through innovative medical and health care technologies, new products, and services. These developments with markets being in the center are leading to increasing turnover, higher revenue and growing profits as a basis for financing other parts of the economy, including the first health sector. In addition, new therapy professions, new study fields and new university research areas are emerging.

As can be seen from a study sponsored by the Robert Bosch Foundation in 2007 [14], reference human capital as a blending of health and education forms one of Germany's most important strategic resources. Its quantity and quality decide how the future will be mastered. Human capital is one of the most important determinants of economic growth. The accumulation of human capital through investments in health and education is crucial for the innovative capacities of a national economy. Both sectors promote the growth of the remaining sectors of the economy, and through their own development they themselves become an essential source of growth.

Within the union of health and education, health is a prerequisite in the service of education. People can only use their human capital effectively if they are healthy and alive. In its Global Development Report 2007 [15], the world bank defined investments in human capital via health and education as the crucial prerequisite for success in today's competitive globalized world, whether as an individual or as an entire economic unit. For most people, employability is the only asset which needs to be made permanently more productive in order to sustain and continually regenerate prosperity. This means learning to make the correct decisions in order to stay healthy and then adhering to them throughout life. With regard to demographic shift healthy life expectancy is gaining more and more importance.

Health and education "spending" is a term which is often used erroneously when really "investment" is meant. Any expenditure which serves to improve effectiveness and create future benefits may be counted as an investment. We therefore propose apportioning investment spending on health and education so that it appears in the national accounts statistics and national budget not as a cost, but as an investment. Spending on health and education would then cease to be treated like consumer spending, becoming entirely cost-effective in the year of consumption and instead, as is customary for investments, would be amortized over several years. This would take into account the fact that several years can elapse between an investment in health and education and the benefits to be reaped from this investment.

Similar to the creation of satellite systems alongside the national accounts statistics, this development should be promoted for health as a growth factor. According to the neoclassical model by [16], increased productivity resulting from technical progress drives on economic growth from outside the model – exogenously.

The human capital theory takes into account both microeconomics and macroeconomics and was initiated by the Nobel Prize winners for Economics, Schultz, 1971 [17], and Becker, 1975 [18]. This theory permits an examination of the prerequisites for determining the economic viability of investments in human knowledge and human competence, that is, in human capital. It identifies various paths leading to the creation of human capital, for example,

- formal school education,
- professional and social educational and vocational training measures, and
- measures for maintaining and promoting health, such as prevention and health checks.

In the 1960s the theoretical model of human capital as an endogenous driving force behind growth was developed by Becker 1975 [18], 1993 [19] and then developed further by Mankiw et al. 1992 [20]. The high significance attributed to human capital compared to fixed capital can be observed from a comparison between the proportion of the gross domestic product (GDP) invested in fixed capital and in human capital in Germany.

In 2003 the gross fixed capital formation in Germany for equipment, buildings and other investments – real capital – amounted to €384.4 thousand million, corresponding to 17.8% of the GDP. The true investment rate is much higher, however, taking into account the spending on human capital which in the national accounts statistics is included as consumption. This expenditure, often commonly called "investment", including by politicians, comprises money for education, research, and science totalling €193.9 thousand million, money for art and culture totalling €0.8 thousand million, and money for health excluding investments and medical research totalling €222.1 thousand million. This means a total investment in human capital of €416.8 thousand million or 19.3% of the GDP in 2003. Table 1 shows the expenditure for real and human capital according to the records of the Federal Office for Statistics in 2003 [21] (Statistisches Bundesamt).

The "investments" in human capital are thus €32 thousand million above those in real capital. The national economic investment rate is thus 37.1% and not the mere 17.8% measured by only taking the gross fixed capital formation into account.

Expanding the concept of investment within the national accounts statistics (SNA) was discussed by the United Nations Statistics Division prior to the last update in 1993. Aspen [22] then presented the majority opinion of his workgroup, according to which expenditure on research and development should also be treated as an investment in the next SNA revision.

According to the SNA, expenditure is an investment if it serves to improve effectiveness or productivity and if it creates future benefits. Expenditure on research and development was attributed these characteristics. In the opinion of the United

Table 1 Expenditure on real and human capital in Germany in 2003, in thousand million Euros

Gross domestic product (GDP)	2163.4
Fixed capital	
Total gross fixed capital formation	384.4
Percentage of GDP	17.8
Human capital	
Expenditure education, research, science	193.9
Expenditure art and culture	0.8
Health-related expenditure excl. investments and med. research	222.1
Total human capital	416.8
Percentage of GDP	19.3

Nations Statistics Division [22], expenditure on human capital has comparable characteristics to that for research and development.

In order to be able to treat expenditure on human capital as an investment in the national accounts statistics, the following problems need to be solved:

- clear criteria for the apportionment of investment spending on human capital
- the investment product must be clearly definable
- the product must be able to be evaluated in an economically reasonable manner
- the amortization rate of the product must be known.

Despite these unsolved problems, the discussion about classifying spending on human capital as an investment will continue. The 1992 Nobel Prize winner for Economics, Gary S. Becker [23], advocates that expenditure on education and health be treated as investments in both the national accounts statistics and tax. Nordhaus [24] and Cuttler [25] also advocate inclusion of health in the national accounts statistics once the methodical problems surrounding this have been solved.

Preventive orientation of health care and consequently the exhaustion of previously unexploited health potential is another as yet unsolved task. According to the latest literature, the key to primary prevention is the avoidance of risk factors for chronic diseases, such as smoking, unhealthy diet, being overweight or obese, failure to take physical exercise, alcohol abuse, and addressing health determinants. Primary prevention is aimed at reducing the probability of the onset of chronic and other diseases. According to the latest literature, over 50% of chronic diseases can be avoided through primary prevention of risk factors.

To date, every significant progressive step related to public health has been connected to improve the determinants of health resulting in the reduction and control of risk factors. The first significant step was the avoidance of risk factors for infectious diseases in the mid-19th century, notably the observance of rules pertaining to hygiene. The next significant step to boost public health will have to be the avoidance of risk factors for chronic diseases [26–28].

Overview of Existing Empirical Evidence

One essential reason why hardly any connection, or only a contradictory one, is ascertainable between health-related spending and a measurable improvement in health is that health-related spending is predominantly measured only according to inputs and not outputs. The research question which needs to be answered is how growth can be assigned to a specific investment health-related outlay. According to provisional estimates by Nordhaus [24], consumptive spending on health over the last 50 years has contributed to prosperity to the same extent as other consumptive spending. Using the current methods of economic evaluation, we are not yet in a position to say whether €1 spent on health has a return which may be €2, 4, or 10 higher than for that spent on other consumer needs.

The literature reporting microeconomic investigations into investments made by firms in the health of their employees is very extensive. Numerous studies in the USA are concerned, for example, with health productivity management (HPM). The results of these studies draw a direct link between the health of employees and their productivity, influencing the profit made by the company and ultimately its share price [29]. Activities are geared toward reducing sick-leave costs and increasing productivity by improving the general health of staff. Example publications include Refs. [30–35].

Bloom [36] investigated whether at a macroeconomic level there is a correlation between health and economic coefficients corresponding to that shown by microeconomic studies. He estimated that an increase of 1% in the adult survival rate results in an increase of approximately 2.8% in labor productivity. In his opinion, health plays a larger role in the promotion of economic growth than education.

Sanso [37] examined the connection between life expectancy and growth. In his opinion the accumulation of human capital and innovative medical techniques permits individual decisions to be made not only about the quality of life, but also about its length. The desire in ageing citizens to counteract biological deterioration in order to maintain a high level of quality of life will in the future become a driving economic force. Medical science and the health care economy will provide techniques and products which slow down the loss of quality of life through the biological ageing process. The state of health of future generations will thus be improved. This will result in increasing individual performance over a longer lifetime, inducing economic growth. According to Sanso [37], this growth will generate sufficient resources to finance medical research and health-related expenditure.

Cutler [38] conducted a study to investigate the value of health-related spending in the United States over a period of 40 years – 1960–2000. The increase in life expectancy in the USA was compared to the costs of illness and disease. In summary he concluded that over the entire 40-year period the cost of one additional year of life expectancy for a newborn baby averaged $19,900. For those aged 65 years and over, the same increase over the same period cost an average of $84,700. One of his essential conclusions is that 70% of the reason for increased life expectancy in newborn babies between 1960 and 2000 is the reduced mortality rate resulting from cardiovascular diseases.

According to [38], the current trends with regard to cost development are worrying, however. Following his calculation, the cost of one additional year of life expectancy increased dramatically in the last two decades of his investigation, especially for the older age groups. His analyses to prove an increase in life expectancy for the over-65 s show that in the 1970s one additional year cost $46,800, whereas by the 1990s this figure had risen to $145,000. The rate of increase for health-related spending per year of extended life expectancy is thus significantly higher than the rate of increase for years of age. If this trend is sustained, Cutler [38] worries that the cost effectiveness of health-related spending for elderly citizens will decrease.

The latest publication on this topic [39] purports the view that investments in health have a significant impact on economic development. A good state of health in a population makes a crucial contribution to the development of human capital and labor productivity. In the opinion of the author, competition is in a position to increase effectiveness, but the state must assume responsibility for just financing and access to essential health care goods. In acknowledging this responsibility, the state could even make a point of increasing health-related expenditure.

Macroeconomics and Health

The recent Report by the WHO Commission on Macroeconomics and Health, chaired by Professor Jeffrey Sachs [40], shows that if world leaders are serious about reducing poverty and fostering development, they have to invest in health. And, in its Report, the Commission showed how health investments can be managed in order to achieve the best results.

A study of the global figures shows that three avoidable diseases; HIV/AIDS, tuberculosis and malaria are overwhelmingly important. Maternal and child conditions, reproductive ill-health, injuries, and the health consequences of tobacco, are also global health priorities. Any serious attempt to reduce the disease burden faced by the world's poorest people must concentrate on all these conditions. Any serious attempt to stimulate global economic and social development, and so to promote human security, must be successful in addressing the burdens caused by AIDS, malaria, and TB.

Of the burden caused by the three diseases, HIV/AIDS makes up just over half, both in terms of healthy life years lost, and mortality. Malaria and TB share the rest on a roughly equal basis. It means that more than 90 million healthy life years are lost to HIV each year, 40 million to malaria and nearly 36 million to TB. More than 5.5million lives are lost every year to the three diseases alone.

One of the latest documents by the Commission of the European Communities is a Commission Staff Working Document accompanying the White Paper: Together for Health – A Strategic Approach for the European Union 2008–2013 [41]. It aims to be a cohesive framework document, giving clear directions for Community activities in the field of health for the coming years, in order to continue to improve and protect health within the EU and beyond its borders. It reinforces the importance of health within key EC policies, such as the Lisbon Strategy for Growth and Jobs reference, in terms of the links between health and economic prosperity, and the Citizen's Agenda, in terms of people's right to be empowered in their health and health care. The strategy is a cross-sectoral framework which recognizes the contribution to health of a wide range of policy areas.

According to the White Paper, there is growing evidence that health contributes to wealth and that investment in health contributes to long-term economic growth and sustainability. Health policy makers have long been arguing, as mentioned already, that "health means wealth", and that a healthy population is necessary for economic productivity and prosperity, not to forget that wealth, particularly in the form of effective investment, in turn supports better health.

The strategy argues that health-related costs are considerable in the EU, but effective investment in health can lead to more efficient health care systems and Social Security schemes, to more people avoiding illness and therefore to greater future financial sustainability. As well as health care treatment, effective prevention programs can also substantially reduce major and chronic diseases. According to the Commission's White Paper there is growing evidence that increased investment in preventive measures could counteract the expected growth in health-related costs and expenditure. If the aged population remains active and in good health, this is positive both for the individual and for the wider economy. If health-specific life expectancy were to evolve, broadly speaking, in line with changes to age-specific life expectancy, then the projected increase in spending on health due to ageing would be halved.

In order to maximize the years of age which are healthy and to achieve healthy ageing, it is important to promote health and to prevent disease throughout life, including tackling health determinants such as diet, physical exercise, alcohol, drug and tobacco consumption, environmental and socioeconomic factors. The health of the working population is the key factor for economic sustainability. The Community initiatives with regard to health and its impact on society support the way we understand and approach health policy, as outlined in Chapter 1. Health itself has become a major economic and social driving force in society, as described in great detail by Surcke et al. [42].

An important contribution regarding the correlation between health and the economy has been made by [42]. In summary, the authors of this European Commission study conclude that investments in health are good for a national economy for the following reasons:

- the labor force potential becomes more productive and can generate a higher income due to an improved state of health
- an improved state of health facilitates a longer working lifetime, a necessity for a population which is becoming older and producing fewer children
- less sick leave is taken and early retirement becomes less prevalent
- greater investments in education pay more dividends in conjunction with an improved state of health and a longer working lifetime, contributing to an increase in productivity

Table 2 Selected studies from SURCKE 2005 [42] on the correlation between health and the national economy

Author	Title	Year	End points	Conclusion	Publication
Surcke M, Urban D	The role of cardiovascular disease in economic growth	2005	Economic growth	Reducing the cardio-vascular mortality of the labor force by 10% causes economic growth to rise by 1%	Mimeo, WHO European Office for Investment for Health and Development, Venice
Weil D	Accounting for the effect of health on economic growth	2004	GDP per capita	State of health explains 19.1% of differences in income between workers	Department of Economics, Brown University, preliminary
Bloom D, Canning D, Sevilla J	Health, worker productivity and economic growth	2002	GDP per capita	A 1% increase in life expectancy increases labor productivity by 1.7%	School of Public Policy and Management, Carnegie Mellon University, Pittsburgh
Arora S	Health, human productivity, and long-term economic growth	2001	GDP	Health improvements over the past 100–125 years increased economic growth in 10 industrialized nations by 30–40%	Journal of Economic History, Vol. 61, No 3, Sept.
Barro R	Health and economic growth	1996	GDP per capita	Increasing life expectancy from 40 to 70 years increased the growth rate in 100 countries by 1.4% p.a. between 1965 and 1990	PAHO: Program on public policy and health, health and human development division

Table 3 Number of practising physicians per 100.000 inhabitants, based on OECD data and calculations by the Federal Office of Statistics

Year	Germany	Netherlands	Norway	Poland	Russia	Spain	Sweden	Switzerland
Number per 100,000 inhabitants								
1980	–	190.72	191.23	–	–	–	220.20	238.85
1985	–	222.15	220.98	196.76	387.09	–	262.10	273.04
1990	299.57	250.55	248.90	214.18	407.04	–	259.17	298.41
1995	306.53	–	295.26	231.74	385.91	247.39	285.62	316.38
2000	326.04	319.34	292.15	220.02	421.27	316.38	307.34	350.99
2001	330.70	327.82	290.29	224.13	420.37	307.53	283.53	351.41
2002	333.61	338.25	330.49	230.35	425.88	290.94	315.90	355.83
2003	336.75	348.47	338.26	229.39	424.56	322.11	317.95	371.55
2004	339.05	360.37	348.29	224.26	422.09	–	324.57	375.42
2005	340.20	371.30	368.29	.	424.63	–	–	389.56

- an improved state of health increases healthy-life expectancy and requires a higher savings rate, e.g. as provision for old age, thus generating the means for a higher rate of investment.

Surcke [42] examined 65 studies about health in all its various guises and their impact on the economy. Table 2 lists five of these studies in summary.

The 65 studies, performed using a wide range of analytical methods, are all in agreement with the latest literature, stating that the health of a population is the determining factor for personal income and economic growth.

Expanding Understanding of Health: The First and the Second Sector for Health Care and for Health

The health care sector has developed to become the health care economy. Alongside the recording of health-related spending, this sector of the economy is interesting from an economic and political point of view for its value added and its impact on employment. In contrast to other branches of industry and sectors of the economy, the significance of the health care economy for the national economy has yet to be grasped. Firstly, there is no generally acknowledged split up of the health care economy within the national accounts statistics, the health care expenditure calculations and the health care staff calculations. This situation also leads to very different prognoses regarding the development of the health care economy.

With a qualitative segregation, a first area usually focuses on prevention and the promotion of healthy living, curative treatment including care with therapies and medicines, rehabilitation, nursing care and palliative medicine. As well as human medicine, this area also includes dental medicine, which is treated very differently in different countries as far as the remuneration of services is concerned, for example,

Switzerland, New Zealand, and Australia on the one hand, and France, Germany, and the Netherlands on the other. Finally, this area can also include sick pay for employees. A first market for health care covers this core area, that is, the health care sector with all its establishments and providers and remunerable services covered by the health insurance companies or a public health service. It also includes all types of extra payments, surgery fees, or excess payable in times of convalescence.

A second market for health covers an extended range of health-related services and goods which are not included in the first market and which are not covered by private or statutory health insurance or by a public health service. A more detailed segregation can be made according to product, service, and business-related characteristics. This area also includes "over-the-counter" purchases in chemists or medical supply shops. To date there is no uniform segregation between the two areas, that is, one agreed upon across Europe

Additional criteria for segregation can be deduced from the health benefits to be gained from goods and services or from the motivation to buy health-related services and the demand for health-related goods. Finally, expenditure for training, research and development must be included, each represented proportionally in one of the two markets. A division used in the German literature employs the following classes [43].

- wholesalers, specialists, and retailers,
- pharmaceuticals industry, health trade professions, medical technology, biotechnology, and gene technology,
- public administration, health insurance, education, business services, organization of the health care economy, research, and development, as well as
- sport, leisure, wellness, tourism, nutrition, and lifestyle.

Even with this division, a subdivision is necessary if the parts belonging to the health care economy are to be clarified.

In a study by Roland Berger, the authors assume that fitness, wellness, functional food, organic foodstuffs, and health tourism all belong to the second market for health care, albeit to different extents [44]. Finally, the international System of Health Accounts also includes services which are relevant to health but only indirectly linked with it, for example, "meals on wheels".

This variety of approaches demonstrates the difficulties involved in agreeing upon a segregation, and the growing significance of regional health care economy also throws up questions regarding a regional segregation of the markets, with their value added and impact on employment [45].

Last but not least, segregation is made even more difficult by the fact that, in the field of public health, the relevance of health is increasingly being signalized in all areas of life, for example, at nursery school, at school, at home, and at sport. [46].

In addition to qualitative segregation, questions also arise pertaining to a quantitative evaluation of various subdivisions within the health care sector. For example, expenditure can be divided up according to the occasioners of expenditure and how they are financed, functionally according to types of service and institutionally

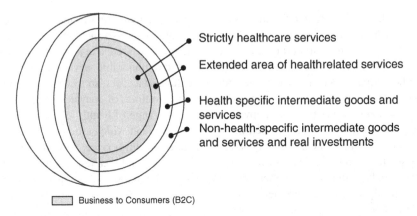

Business to Consumers (B2C)

Fig. 1 Different areas of the health care sector

according to types of establishment. Manpower calculations for the health care sector are also determined by the type of segregation chosen. In this field the workforce in Germany, for example, fluctuates between 4.3 and 4.9 million employees [47].

Against this background of segregating the two markets in different possible ways, evaluations of the impact of employment and the value added also differ for the health care sector.

In one strategy the following proposal has been made for segregating the various areas [48]:

- a core area of strictly health care services, restricted to services covered by health insurance (Bismarck System) or a public health service (Beveridge System)
- an extended area of health-related services covering not only services which are paid for privately, but also expenditure on health-related training and research
- an area of health-specific intermediate goods and services, to include many medical products and characterized by the fact that they are not intended for the end user (business to consumer), but for other manufacturers (business to business)
- a fourth area covering intermediate goods and services in the health care sector not specific to health, e.g. facility management in hospitals, canteen services, laundry services or new building works.

To summarize, the following overview (Fig. 1) illustrates the different areas of the health care sector subject to observation:

Labor Market Implications

In the discussion about segregating the different markets for health care, we mentioned not only expenditure, value added and the impact on employment, but also health care employees. According to the calculations of the Federal Office of

Statistics, in 2004, 10.6% of all employees in Germany were working in the health care sector. Health care employees can be divided up into professions, establishments, and type of employment.

In addition, we can compare the number of practising physicians per 100,000 inhabitants, based on OECD data and calculations by the Federal Office of Statistics.

It should be noted that this comparison ignores important features such as the age structure or morbidity of the individual populations, as well as the age structure or employment structure (number of full-time, part-time, and marginally employed) of the practising physicians. As far as new professions in health care is concerned, there are some important developments not shown in the statistics above [49].

In addition to the two financial advantages for the first health care market resulting from the expanding second market (see above), other desirable effects are also emerging in the light of the demographic development and the many technological innovations. The older population, in many countries not suffering from poverty, is demanding new products and services in connection with sickness and health, and with this increasing demand for health-related services numerous changes are occurring in the many labor markets within the health care sector.

New vocational training and professional opportunities are changing qualification requirements and existing job descriptions, for example, in nursing, nutritional expertise, management and information technology, or medical engineering. The physician's assistant, the study nurse, the nurse practitioner, the surgical-technical assistant, the orthoptist, the tele-nurse, and the patient scout are all new occupations, some of which require academic training. These positions all serve to guide patients, their families and insured parties more easily through the highly complex health care system, with its still predominantly sectoral services and their fragmented financing and intransparent remuneration. Linked to this change there are also new areas of work in research and development.

The staff-intensive health care field is, therefore, also a growth industry, with the expansion of existing employment opportunities and the development of new job descriptions [50]. Bearing this in mind, public discussion about the so-called cost explosion and the linked nonwage labor costs needs to be reassessed (see above). The latter can be reduced through new financing options, but even an increase in health care expenditure financed by wages and salaries has a stronger multiplicative effect on growth than rising pension-related expenditure [51].

We have already addressed the impact of the second sector for health care on professions within the health care sector. One peculiarity consists in the fact that these new job descriptions cannot usually be obviously assigned to one market or the other. Ambulatory nursing services are also individually available, independently of nursing care and health insurance stipulations, and physiotherapists, as well as other service providers, are happy to do business with patients directly.

Aside from these examples of a financing mix for health care services combining insurance cover and private payments, and thus of a financing of services from different sources, the labor market will experience further innovations. In the light of the current demographic development, the rise in chronic diseases and the increasing support required by the elderly in this context will lead to increased health care expenditure. This concerns not only the health care services traditionally covered by statutory health and nursing care insurance, but also the help required in later life, and thus new services. More and more people are living alone and require support at home in order to continue to do so, and in this field the abovementioned and other job descriptions will undergo a dynamic development.

A stronger inclusion of nonmedical health care professions within the health care sector means that increasing importance will be attached to staff qualifications. In the field of wellness, for example, it is becoming increasingly difficult for consumers to differentiate between serious providers and less good services. It should be emphasized that there is a real need for quality assurance through well-trained staff, especially in conjunction with the care of older and geriatric patients – for example, with degenerative diseases. For this increasingly significant target group, dubious, and unqualified providers of health-related services can even represent a danger to health.

Structures within the vocational training system need to take these developments on board flexibly and quickly. This also concerns a redistribution of tasks within a professional world which is changing through telecommunication, the alleviation of manual tasks through technical intervention, as well as work in new teams [52]. The telemedical care of patients with chronic cardiac insufficiency, and joint data documentation are also part of this new development, as well as a new orientation of nonmedical fields such as speech therapy, physiotherapy, hospital logistics, or nursing science in general. Freelancing must also be possible. Last but not least, the Internet has meant profound changes to the all-important patient–physician relationship [53]. This development shows that the impact of the second market for health care will mean changes in job distribution, as well as a specialization of the services provided and their quality assurance. In the light of this foreseeable development it would be desirable to have everyone working with and not against one another.

On the Growth-Related Effects of Health Promotion

A good health economics scenario analysis of the potential economic impact of prevention is the report by Wanless [54, 55]. The author was requested by the Chancellor of the Exchequer to investigate the long-term trends which could shape the British health care system (National Health Service, NHS) in the next 20 years. His strategy was that health care would gain such economic significance as to become a dynamic force not only responsible for producing a healthy population and a healthy workforce, but also promoting employment and national prosperity in its own right. Prevention and a healthy lifestyle would both play major roles. Three different strategic scenarios were selected to demonstrate cost development between 2002 and 2023.

Scenario 1: Solid progress. People become more engaged in relation to their health: life expectancy rises considerably, health status improves and people have confidence in the primary care system and use it more appropriately. The health service is responsive with high rates of technology uptake and a more efficient use of resources.

Scenario 2: Slow uptake. There is no change in the level of public engagement: life expectancy rises by the lowest amount in all three scenarios and the health status of the population is constant or deteriorates. The health service is relatively unresponsive with low rates of technology uptake and low productivity.

Scenario 3: Fully engaged. Levels of public engagement in relation to their health are high: life expectancy increases go beyond current forecasts, health status improves dramatically and people are confident in the health system and demand high-quality care. The health service is responsive with high rates of technology uptake, particularly in relation to disease prevention. Use of resources is more efficient.

Table 4 shows expenditure on health care in Britain (National Health Service, NHS) relative to GDP for the period 2002 to 2023 according to the three scenarios proposed by Wanless [55].

As is the case with all scenario analyses, the results are sensitive to the assumptions upon which they are based. In the "Solid progress" scenario, health-related expenditure relative to GDP rises to 11.1% by 2023. Should, however, the increase in productivity within the health care sector fall just 1% short of that assumed in the scenario, with all other factors remaining the same, expenditure relative to GDP would increase to 13.1%. Vice versa, a 1% improvement in productivity compared to the assumed level in 2023, with all other factors remaining the same, would mean a lower expenditure relative to GDP of 9.4%. This finding underlines the necessity of health care reforms in order to achieve desired targets.

The scenario "Fully engaged" is the least expensive and yet boasts better results than the other two scenarios, not least because of its preventive orientation. According to Wanless [55], the state of the population's health would improve by considerably reducing major risk factors such as smoking, obesity, poor diet, and insufficient physical exercise. The percentage of smokers would then be close to that found in California today. Following the assumptions of the scenario "Fully engaged", this reduction in risk factors would be at its greatest where they are currently to be found most often, namely in the parts of the population with the lowest social standing.

In addition to considerably reducing major risk factors, the scenario "Fully engaged" aims to develop from a "system of sickcare" into a "system of health

Table 4 Expenditure on health care in Britain relative to GDP (in %) in three different scenarios set out in the Wanless Report

Scenario	2002	2007–2008	2012–2013	2017–2018	2022–2023
Solid progress	7.7	9.4	10.5	10.9	11.1
Slow uptake	7.7	9.5	11.0	11.9	12.5
Fully engaged	7.7	9.4	10.3	10.6	10.6

care", in which healthy people can remain fit and those with chronic diseases can remain as active as possible. The lower expenditure resulting from this optimistic scenario compared to the other two is explained as follows.

Spending increases as the result of a growing population with a higher life expectancy making more use of outpatient treatment for preventive care and counselling purposes. This is counteracted by savings, estimated to be greater than the increase in spending, chiefly resulting from a reduction in the prevalence of geriatric diseases and an improvement to the general state of health in the population through prevention. Expenditure in scenario 3 "Fully engaged" is £30 thousand million or approximately 20% lower for 2023 than in scenario 2 "Slow uptake".

For the growth potential of a national economy, development of the labor force potential, as well as the workers activated from this potential in order to generate the GDP, are more important than the overall development of the population [56].

The reality in the German labor market is that the average working life ends aged 60. Few workers today reach the legally stipulated retirement age of 65 years, which is why the average for both men and women is around 60 years. On 01.02.2006 a new law was passed to raise the retirement age to 67 years by 2029. It will be raised in gradual steps, starting in 2012. However, the labor force which is currently actually available has a prevailing age range of 20–60 years and disregards the official retirement age of 65, not to mention that of 67 envisaged for 2029.

This leads researchers to question how prevention-orientated health care could succeed in raising the real age limit of the labor force potential from its current 60 years to a possible 70 years by 2050. This extension of employment age to 70 years was recommended, for example, by the German Institute for Economic Research in 2005 [57].

Table 5 assumes for its minimum and maximum variants in its 2002 line that the actual age limit remains the same between 2002 and 2050, even if a higher retirement age is stipulated by law (20–65, 20–70).

Table 5 Development from 2002 to 2050 of the labor force potential aged 20–60, 20–65, 20–70 years based on 1000 persons and in accordance with two variants by the Federal Office of Statistics 2006 [58] compared to Basis 2002

	20–60	20–65	20–70
Variant 1: minimum variant – potential labor force by age group			
2002	45,354	45,354	45,354
2050	29,901	34,834	39,468
Difference	−15,453	−10,520	−5886
Variant 2: maximum variant – potential labor force by age group			
2002	45,354	45,354	45,354
2050	35,240	40,540	45,466
Difference	−10,114	−4814	112

The column differences for the minimum and maximum variants show how the labor force potential would develop by 2050, compared to the baseline year 2002, simply by changing its age range from 20–60 years to 20–65 years to 20–70 years.

In the scenario with the minimum variant the labor force potential in the column 20–60 drops 15.5 million persons by 2050.

Increasing the actual age range to 20–65 years would reduce the labor force potential by 10.5 million persons, and a range of 20–70 years would reduce it by just 5.9 million.

The maximum variant also assumes in its 2002 line that the actual age limit remains the same between 2002 and 2050, even if a higher retirement age is stipulated (20–65, 20–70). In this scenario the labor force potential in the column 20–60 years drops 10.1 million persons by 2050.

Increasing the actual age range to 20–65 years would reduce the labor force potential by just 4.8 million persons and increasing it to 20–70 years would even induce a slight increase of 0.112 million.

Comparing the minimum and maximum variants with the different age limits, the most favorable variant – accepting the assumptions of the Federal Office of Statistics – turns out to be the combination of a real age range of 20–70 years with the maximum variant for population development until 2050. The assumptions of the Federal Office of Statistics comprise a slight increase in the birth rate from 1.4 to 1.6 children per woman capable of child-bearing, a high life expectancy and a net migration of 200,000 persons per annum. Accordingly, in 2050 the labor force potential would still have approximately the same level it had in 2002, despite an overall reduction in the population.

Raising the retirement age by law is not in itself enough to achieve a significant increase in labor force potential. Without improving the state of health of the population, raising the retirement age will primarily induce pension cuts. The labor force potential consists only of the population at employable age, for example, 20–70 years, and contains the subset of workers generating the income for nonworkers throughout the population and across all age groups.

The process by which the labor force potential is rendered capable of generating the GDP is influenced by many factors, of which health is only one. According to SIDDAL 2007, the reasons given for early retirement by 55–64 year olds in 15 EU states were health-related in up to 25% of cases. In Germany the percentage is 22.9.

According to the report Gesundheit in Deutschland (Health in Germany) [59], chronic diseases are the most frequent cause of early retirement and include skeletal, muscular, and connective tissue disorders; circulatory disorders; psychiatric disorders; and carcinogenic diseases. Together these four disease groups were the cause of early retirement in 78% of women and 75% of men in 2003.

The, Director of the Office of Behavioral and Social Sciences Research of the National Institutes of Health in the USA [60], ascertained the following in celebration of the 10th anniversary of his Office on 15th June 2006: approximately 70% of our state of health is attributable to individual, group and social behavior, representing social determinants.

It would exceed the scope of this chapter to provide a model calculation for how an actual raising of the retirement age and a prevention-orientated health care system, achieved through investments in human capital and a realization of the assumptions for increasing labor productivity by 2050, could affect economic growth and the financing of income and social services. Future investigations into the economic impact of a higher value added potential through investments in human capital should address the following theories, to name but a few:

- The Social Security contribution rates are increasing more slowly than previously assumed or not at all since the growing expenditure predicted as a result of demographic change and medical progress can be financed by the national insurance systems at no extra cost through constant deductions from higher income.
- With the labor force potential weakened by demographic change, the high stake held in world trade by Germany and the EU can still be maintained if labor productivity is considerably increased.
- Because of the high investments in human capital necessary to safeguard a high value added potential, if the labor force potential is continually to reproduce it must have at its disposal an income which only a highly productive, high-wage economy can finance. A high value added potential cannot be guaranteed with low wage levels in the long term.

In order to assert itself, a national strategy for growth and jobs requires human capital which is equal in quality to the human capital of its competitors, or better still superior. This can only be realized by investing in human capital as the union of health and education. Once achieved, this then generates a good basis for adopting policies to create a highly productive, high-wage economy.

References

1. Health at a Glance 2007, OECD Indicators – ISBN 978-92-64-02732-9 – OECD 2007.
2. US Department of Health and Human Services "Leading Health Indicators Selected for Healthy People 2010" or the "Main Categories for the European Community Health Indicators Set" or the costs of disease, e.g. for Germany in 2004. Federal Office of Statistics.
3. Zimmermann, H., Henke, K.-D., Finanzwissenschaft, 9th edition, Munich 2005, pp. 93–108.
4. Hernandez Aguado in this volume.
5. Special Report 1996 and Special Report 1997 (*both in German*), Healthcare in Germany, Cost Factor and Future Industry, Vol I: Demography, Morbidity, Economic Reserves and Employment, and Vol II: Progress and Growth Markets, Financing and Remuneration, Baden-Baden 1996 and Baden-Baden 1997/98.
6. Neubauer, G. From national insurance to healthcare economy, in Adam, H., et al., eds., Public Finances and Healthcare Economy, Baden-Baden 2007, pp. 200 (*in German*).
7. The healthcare economy, Das Journal für die Akteure der Gesundheitsbranche, Nr. 1, February/March 2008 (*in German*).
8. Henke, K.-D., Cobbers, B., Georgi, A., Schreyögg, J., Berlin's healthcare economy – growth and employment prospects, 2nd edition, Berlin 2006; Kartte, J., et al., Innovation and growth in the healthcare system, Roland Berger View, Berlin, no year; Hilbert, J., Healthcare metropolis Ruhr, growth opportunities and development potential of the healthcare economy, 2005;

Healthcare City Berlin e.V., ed., Healthcare economy, competences and prospects of the region around the capital – a manual, Berlin 2007 (*in German*).

9. World Health Organization, ed., Macroeconomics and Health: Investing in Health for Economic Development, Report of the Commission on Macroeconomics and Health, chaired by Jeffrey D. Sachs, Genf 2001 and WHO, Increasing Investments in Health Outcomes for the Poor, 2nd Consultation on Macroeconomics and Health, Genf 2003, as well as sowie Pogge, T., Growth and Inequality: Understanding Recent Trends and Political Choices, in Dissent Megazine, dissentmagazine.org/article/?article = 990.

10. European Commission, Health & Consumer Protection, Directorate – General, The Contribution of Health to the Economy of the European Union, Luxemburg 2005.

11. Nolte, E., Scholz, R., Shkolmikov, V., Mc Kee, M. (2002) The contribution of medical care to changing life expectancy in Germany and Poland, Soc Sci Med 55: 1905–1921.

12. Byrne, D., Health equals wealth, speech held on the European Health Forum, Bad Gastein, 2003, europa.eu.int/rapid/start/cgi/guesten.ksh?p˙action.getfile = gf&doc = SPEECH/03/443/ = /AGED&Ig = EN = type = PDF, download November, 15 2003.

13. Henke, K.-D., Health as a Macroeconomic Driver – The health market and its contribution to productivity and economic growth, 9th European Health Forum Gastein 2006, Partnerships for Health.

14. Martin K., Henke K.D. (2007) Gesundheitsökonomische Szenarien zur Prävention, sponsored by the Robert Bosch Foundation, Stuttgart.

15. World Bank (2007) World Development Report and the Next Generation. The World Bank Group, Washington.

16. Solow R.M. (1956) A contribution to the theory of economic growth. Q J Econ 70(1): 65–94.

17. Schultz T.Z. (1971) Investment in Human Capital. The Free Press, Chicago.

18. Becker G.S. (1975) Human Capital. Chicago University Press, Chicago.

19. Becker G.S. (1993) Human Capital: A Theoretical and Empirical Analysis, with Special Reference to Education, 3rd edition. The University of Chicago Press, Chicago.

20. Mankiw N.G. et al. (1992) A contribution to the empirics of economic growth. Q J Econ 107(2): 407–437.

21. Statistisches Bundesamt (2003) Bevölkerungsentwicklung Deutschlands von 2002 bis 2050. Ergebnisse der 10. koordinierten Bevölkerungsvorausberechnung, Wiesbaden.

22. Aspen C. (1993) Update of the SNA-Issue No. 9 and 10. Issue paper for the meeting of the AEG, July 2005. Extending the asset boundary to include research and development. United Statistics Division, SNA/M1.05/20.

23. Becker G.S. (1996) Human capital: one investment where America is way ahead. Business Week, March 11.

24. Nordhaus W.D. (2002) The Health of Nations: The contribution of improved health to Living Standards. Cowles Foundation for Research in Economics, Yale University, New Haven.

25. Cutler D., Richardson E. (1997) Measuring the health of the US population. Brookings Papers on Economic Activity: Microeconomics, 217–271.

26. WHO (2002) The World Health Report. Reducing Risks, Promoting Healthy Life, Geneva.

27. WHO (2008) Prevention and control of noncommunicable diseases: implementation of the global strategy. Report by the Secretariat, EB122/9, Geneva.

28. Wiener G. et al. (2003) Multimorbidität in Deutschland. Stand – Entwicklung – Folgen. Robert Koch-Institut, Berlin.

29. Goetzel R.Z. (1999) Employee Health and Productivity. Vice President and Director of Consulting and National Practice. The MEDSTAT Group Inc.

30. Riedel et al. (2001) The effect of disease prevention and health promotion on workplace productivity: a literature review. Am J Health Promot, Jan/Feb.

31. Goetzel R.Z., Ozminkowski R.J. (2000) Health and productivity management: emerging opportunities for health promotion professionals for the 21st century. Am J Health Promot, Mar/Apr.

32. Poole S.W. et al. (2001) The impact of an incentive-based worksite health promotion program on modifiable health risk factors. Am J Health Promot, Sep/Oct.

33. Eriksen M.P., Gottlieb N.H. (1998) A review of the health impact of smoking control at the workplace. Am J Health Promot, Nov/Dec.

34. Grosch J.W. et al. (1998) Worksite health promotion programs in the US: factors associated with availability and participation. Am J Health Promot, Sep/Oct.

35. Heany C.A., Goetzel R.Z. (1997) A review of health-related outcomes of multi-component worksite health promotion programs. Am J Health Promot, Mar/Apr.

36. Bloom et al. (2002) Health, worker productivity and economic growth. School of Public Policy and Management, Carnegie Mellon University, Pittsburgh.

37. Sanso M., Rosa M.A. (2006) Endogenous longevity, biological deterioration and economic growth. J Health Econ; 25/3: 555–578.

38. Cutler D.M. (2006) The value of medical spending in the United States, 1960–2000. N Engl J Med; 355: 920–927.

39. Heller P.S. (2007) What should macroeconomists know about Health Care Policy? IMF Working Paper No. 07/13.

40. WHO (no year) Investing in Health. A Summary of the Findings of the Commission on Macroeconomics and Health. CMH Support Unit, Geneva.

41. European Commission (2007) Commission Staff Working Document accompanying the White Paper: Together for Health – A Strategic Approach for the European Union 2008–2013, Brussels.

42. Surcke M. et al. (2005) The contribution of Health to the economy in the European Union. European Commission, Health and Consumer Protection Directorate-General, Luxemburg Office for Official Publications of the European Communities.

43. Hilbert et al. Rahmenbedingungen und Herausforderungen der Gesundheitswirtschaft, Gelsenkirchen 2002.

44. Kartte, J., Neumann, K., Kainzinger, F., Henke, K.-D., Innovation und Wachstum im Gesundheitswesen, Roland Berger View, November 2005.

45. Case study on Berlin's healthcare economy.

46. Stähl, T., et al., Health in All Policies – Prospects and Potentials, Finnish Ministry of Social Affairs and Health, 2006.

47. Federal Office of Statistics (2006) Gesundheit – Ausgaben, Krankheitskosten und Personal 2004, pp. 41, and the study Entwicklungspotentiale der Gesundheitswirtschaft in Niedersachsen (2003) BASYS, NIW, pp. 119.

48. Roland Berger Strategy Consultants, Berlin University of Technology (Financial Science and Healthcare Economics), BASYS GmbH, Erstellung eines Satellitenkontos für die Gesundheitswirtschaft in Deutschland, Forschungsangebot, Berlin 2008, pp. 15.

49. The following section is based on parts of a published text. Henke, K.-D., Neue Berufe im zweiten Gesundheitsmarkt, in Public Health Forum, in press.

50. Henke, K.-D., Cobbers, B., Georgi, A., Schreyögg, J., Die Berliner Gesundheitswirtschaft – Perspektiven für Wachstum und Beschäftigung, 2nd edition. MVW, Berlin 2006.

51. Sachverständigenrat für die Konzertierte Aktion im Gesundheitswesen, Sondergutachten 1996, Gesundheitswesen in Deutschland, Kostenfaktor und Zukunftsbranche, Vol I: Demographie, Morbidität, Wirtschaftlichkeitsreserven und Beschäftigung, Baden-Baden 1996, pp. 235–266.

52. Vgl. Sachverständigenrat Gesundheit (2007) Kooperation und Verantwortung – Voraussetzungen einer zielorientierten Gesundheitsversorgung, Bonn, S. 137 sowie Höppner, K., Stärkere Einbeziehung nicht-ärztlicher Gesundheitsberufe in die Gesundheitsversorgung, in: Die Ersatzkasse, Heft 10/2007, S. 393–396 aber auch Rabbata, S., "Ärztliche Verantwortung ist nicht teilbar", in Deutsches Ärzteblatt, Jg. 104, Heft 44, 2. November 2007, S. A 2988 sowie Lohmann, H., Lohfert, Chr., Medizin im Zentrum des Umbruchs. Erfolgsfaktoren im Überlebenskampf der Krankenhäuser, Hamburg 2007.

53. Siehe Henke, K.-D., Zehn Thesen zur Arzt-Patienten-Beziehung aus gesund-heitswirtschaftlicher Sicht, in: Schumpelick, V., Vogel, B., Hrsg., Arzt und Patient. Eine Beziehung im Wandel, Freiburg im Breisgau 2006, S. 115–124.
54. Wanless D (2002) Securing our future health: taking a long-term view. Final Report. The Public Enquiry Unit, HM Treasury, Parliament Street, London.
55. Wanless D (2004) Securing Health for the Whole Population. Final Report, HM Treasury, London.
56. Deutsche Bank Research (2003) Aktuelle Themen, Demografie Spezial. Deutsches Wachs-tumspotenzial: Vor demographischer Herausforderung, Nr. 277, Frankfurt am Main.
57. Deutsches Institut für Wirtschaftsforchung (2005). Handlungsbedarf. ZDF und Tagesspiegel.
58. Statistisches Bundesamt (2006) Bevölkerungsentwicklung Deutschlands bis 2050. Ergebnisse der 11. koordinierten Bevölkerungsvorausberechnung, Presseexemplar, Wiesbaden.
59. Gesundheit in Deutschland (2006) Kommission Gesundheitsberichterstattung, Abteilung Epidemiologie und Gesundheitsberichterstattung des Robert Koch Instituts, Gruppe Gesund-heit des Statistischen Bundesamtes. Gesundheit in Deutschland – Gesundheitsberichterstat-tung des Bundes, Berlin.
60. Abrams D (2006) Office of Behavioral and Social Sciences, National Institutes of Health.

Berlin's Health care Market as a Driving Economic Force: A Regional Case Study

Abstract

Berlin's health care economy is a continually growing market with potentials which are increasingly attracting attention. The following is an endeavor to demonstrate the significance of Berlin's health care market as a branch of industry, using quantitative parameters. Trends and structural changes over the last few years are particularly visible in the development of turnover and employment. The prospects for growth and employment in Berlin's health care economy become especially clear in a comparison with other branches of industry. Against this background it is important that Berlin be expanded as a centre of science, industry and medical care[1].

Turnover and Gross Value Added of Berlin's Health care Market

A market analysis of Berlin as a health care region requires not only an analysis of the demand for health-related services, but also an examination of its supply structures. The baseline economic situation can be characterized using two coefficients – turnover and gross value added. The overall turnover of Berlin's health care market is the sum of the turnover of all its submarkets. In 2004 this was approximately €14.1 thousand million, 19.8% higher than the turnover in 2000, totalling €11.8 thousand million. The supply side results from a division of Berlin's health care economy into seven different submarkets, each with its respective turnover (cf. Fig. 1). A clear observation is that industry, i.e. the medical technology industry and the pharmaceuticals industry, is responsible for more than half the growth, followed by the hospitals, retail and trade, as well as ambulatory care. Figure 1 also shows the turnover development of the individual submarkets compared to 2000.

In addition to turnover, a second output compilation coefficient describing the performance of a national economy is gross value added. If the intermediate goods and services which occur in the creation of products and services are deducted from the overall turnover, the result is the gross value added and thus the contribution of a branch of industry to the gross national income of an individual economy. However, the concessions are difficult to quantify due to their intersectoral and intrasectoral overlap. Because of this, in 1996 the Committee of Experts for the Concerted Action in Healthcare assumed a 40% deduction when evaluating gross value added for the German health care market [1, 2]. Following the assumption that the production structure with regard to production levels and concessions across the whole of

---

[1] This case study has already been published in German. See Georgi, A., Henke, K.-D., Die Berliner Gesundheitswirtschaft: Zahlen, Daten, Fakten, Strategien, in: Gesundheitsstadt Berlin e.V:, ed., Handbuch Gesundheitswirtschaft, Kompetenzen und Perspektiven der Hauptstadtregion, Berlin 2007, pp. 498–503. An earlier version in English was published in 2004 [11]. A similar regional study was conducted by Neubauer, G., Lewis, P. for Munich [13].

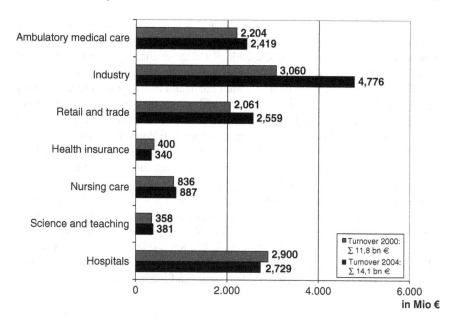

Fig. 1 Comparison of turnover for Berlin's health care economy submarkets between the years 2000 and 2004, own compilation
Source: Henke K-D, Cobbers B, Georgi A, Schreyögg J (2006), Die Berliner Gesundheitswirtschaft – Perspektiven für Wachstum und Beschäftigung, 2nd edition, Berlin 2006, p. 95

Germany cannot be so different from that in Berlin, this figure can be transferred for our purposes. For 2004 this means an estimated gross value added of approximately €8.5 thousand million for Berlin's health care economy. This in turn corresponds to 11.6% of the gross value added for all areas of Berlin's economy in the same year. In comparison, health care across the whole of Germany is only responsible for approximately 4–5% of gross value added [1–3]. In view of the higher density of health care establishments in urban regions, the figure evaluated for Berlin comes as no surprise; indeed, it illuminates the considerable importance of the health care market in Berlin.

The growth of the health care market reflects a shift in consumer preferences, with the increased use of health-related services frequently corresponding to an increased need for services [12]. It should not be ignored, however, that the effect on demand of altered preferences for health-related services is probably very distorted due to tight regulation. A growing health care market strengthens the growth of a society and should therefore be regarded as positive, as long as the rising nonwage labor costs resulting from increasing health insurance premiums do not represent a regional disadvantage.

Health-Related Spending in the Capital

The increase in health-related spending means a wealth of new jobs in related areas. This trend is also noticeable in Berlin (cf. section 'Employment potential in the

Berlin region'). The exact expenditure for health care in the capital has not been explicitly identified, however. The figure can be estimated by taking into consideration the calculation made by the Federal Office of Statistics for health-related spending in 2003, whereby the statutory and private health insurance companies were together responsible for 65.4% of national health care expenditure in Germany [4]. Taking the expenditure of the statutory and private health insurance companies in Berlin as a basis, namely €5.1 thousand million, and assuming that this sum represents 65.4% of Berlin's health-related spending, it follows that total expenditure would be €7.9 thousand million. This means that, in total, an estimated €7.9 thousand million is spent in Berlin by the various occasioners of health-related expenditure on services, premiums and other payments.

In 2004, Berlin's gross domestic product was €77.9 thousand million, approximately 10.1% of which was health-related expenditure [5]. Compared with the national average for health of 10.6% in 2004, Berlin's spending in this area would be slightly less according to this estimate. Taken alongside the comparatively high value added percentage for the health care economy on the supply side, this indicates a relatively high external demand (national and international).

Employment Potential in the Berlin Region

Employment in Germany's national economy is influenced by the health care economy in three different ways. By providing health-related services, this sector improves human capital and thus helps to increase productivity [1, 6]. Since in the German health care system employers participate in premium payments through their employers' contribution and thus also in the financing of the statutory health insurance system, its development therefore also affects the level of nonwage labor costs. Finally, a large proportion of employees paying national insurance work in the health care sector. For 2004 the Federal Office of Statistics calculated 4.2 million employees in health-related areas (health care workers and their jobs). In Germany one in nine persons in active employment works in the health care sector.

The picture in Berlin is slightly different. Data from 2004 show approximately 180,000 persons employed in health-related areas, corresponding to 11.7% of the population, or one in eight persons in the capital in active employment [7]. Whereas in Germany approximately 67% of the actively employed work in service occupations, in Berlin the figure for this sector is 84.6%. Since the health care market can predominantly be characterized as a service market, these figures illustrate the importance of the health care market for Berlin's labor market (cf. Fig. 2). The ambulatory field in particular, including dental surgeries, psychotherapists, ergotherapists, speech therapists, homeopathic practitioners, etc., is the most prominent employer in Berlin's health care market, totalling 52,281 employees. The hospitals come in second, with 39,792 employees, and outpatient and in-patient nursing homes and services employ a total of 29,791 persons. It should be noted here that many citizens within Berlin's health care economy work on a voluntary

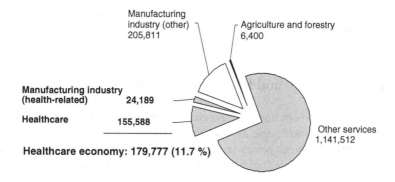

Total number of actively employed: 1,533,500

Fig. 2 Active employment in the different sectors of the Berlin labor market in 2004, own calculation
Source: Henke K-D, Cobbers B, Georgi A, Schreyögg J (2006), Die Berliner Gesundheitswirtschaft – Perspektiven für Wachstum und Beschäftigung, 2nd edition, Berlin 2006, p. 103

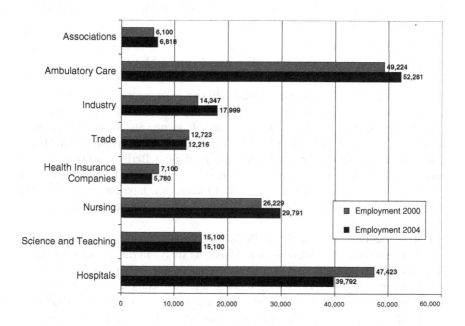

Total employment 2004: 179,777   11.7% of Berlin's gainfully employed

Fig. 3 Comparison of employment rates in the submarkets of Berlin's health care economy between 2000 and 2004
Source: Henke K-D, Cobbers B, Georgi A, Schreyögg J (2006), Die Berliner Gesundheitswirtschaft – Perspektiven für Wachstum und Beschäftigung, 2nd edition, Berlin 2006, p. 106

basis, for example, in hospices. A lack of data means that they cannot be quantitatively accounted for, however (cf. Fig. 3).

Monitoring Growth and Employment in Berlin

Following this analysis of turnover and employment, the two coefficients can now be represented in context using monitoring techniques. This presupposes that sufficient data from different points in time are available in order to demonstrate a potential trend. In Fig. 4 one point represents a submarket for a particular year with the coordinates turnover and employment.

Worthy of notice is the pronounced horizontal development of the pharmaceuticals industry in Berlin. The employment rate in this submarket has hardly changed at all since 1995, and yet the turnover has more than doubled. Similar developments can be seen for the pharmacies. A different trend can be observed for in-patient nursing care. Here the development is vertical, that is, employment increased while the turnover remained more or less the same. In contrast, outpatient care experienced remarkable movements in both employment and turnover between 1997 and 2004. The analysis of growth and turnover in Berlin's health care economy is a good instrument for visualizing trends (cf. Fig. 4).

Berlin – An Expanding Health Care Metropolis

Progress in medical technology, coupled with our demographic development, will lead to an increased requirement for personnel, especially in nursing care and outpatient medical care [7, 8]. The high density of science and vocational training, industry, and hospitals in Berlin additionally provides favorable regional conditions. Centres of competence and care networks are developing. Berlin's health care economy as a staff-intensive branch of the services industry is very high-tech, boasting a thriving pharmaceuticals industry, medical technology, biotechnology, and gene technology, as well as research into medical care, information technology, consulting, and software services.

Complementing the "Healthcare Region Berlin-Brandenburg" master plan, the conclusions and recommendations drawn from the study "Berlin's Healthcare Economy" and the comparable study for Brandenburg should support political decision making in the future [7, 9]. Among other things, this would also mean access to an analysis of strengths and weaknesses or a comparison of regional advantages and disadvantages for potential providers, which would make it easier to draw up concepts for developing Berlin's health care market further.

For example, health care technologies could be marketed internationally with the label "Made in Berlin" [7, 10]. Health care brand names will become increasingly important in Germany. Sustained growth is, however, only possible if an intelligent political framework can be put into place. With regard to regional competition,

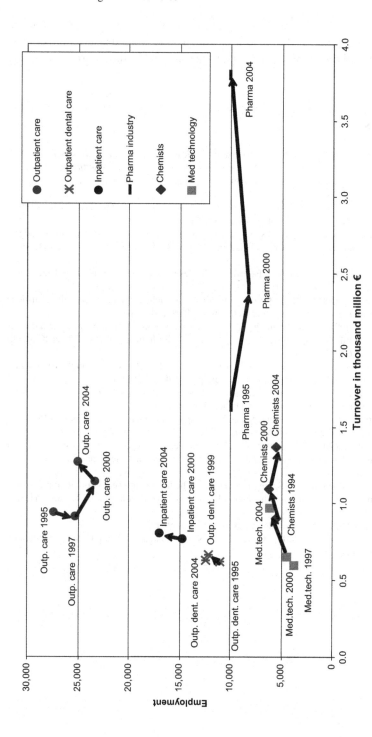

Fig. 4 Development of growth and employment in Berlin's health care economy

Source: Henke K-D, Cobbers B, Georgi A, Schreyögg J (2006), Die Berliner Gesundheitswirtschaft – Perspektiven für Wachstum und Beschäftigung, 2nd edition, Berlin 2006, p. 104

national powers should distance themselves even more from the provision of health care services: what is needed right now is more market and a strong state. The state needs to enforce the economic rules of play, but should then refrain from interfering in the game.

References

1. Sachverständigenrat für die Konzertierte Aktion im Gesundheitswesen (1996), Sondergutachten 1996, Gesundheitswesen in Deutschland – Kostenfaktor und Zukunftsbranche, Bd. I – Demographie, Morbidität, Wirtschaftlichkeitsreserven und Beschäftigung, Baden-Baden.
2. Sachverständigenrat für die Konzertierte Aktion im Gesundheitswesen (1997), Sondergutachten 1997, Gesundheitswesen in Deutschland – Kostenfaktor und Zukunftsbranche, Bd. II: Fortschritt, Wachstumsmärkte, Finanzierung und Vergütung, Baden-Baden.
3. Statistisches Bundesamt (2006), Statistisches Jahrbuch 2005 für die Bundesrepublik Deutschland, Wiesbaden.
4. Statistisches Bundesamt (2005), Fachserie 12, Gesundheitswesen, Ausgaben 1992–2003, Wiesbaden.
5. Statistisches Landesamt Berlin (2005), Statistischer Bericht P I 1-j04, Volkswirtschaftliche Gesamtrechnung und Erwerbstätigenrechnung für Berlin, Berlin.
6. Henke K-D (1999), Beschäftigung in der Dienstleistungs- und Informationsgesellschaft unter besonderer Berücksichtigung des Gesundheitssektors, Beihefte der Zeitschrift für Konjunkturpolitik 48: 63–76.
7. Henke K-D, Cobbers B, Georgi A, Schreyögg J (2006), Die Berliner Gesundheitswirtschaft – Perspektiven für Wachstum und Beschäftigung, 2. Auflage, Berlin.
8. Henke K-D, Reimers L (2005), Finanzierung, Vergütung und Integrierte Versorgung im medizinisch-technischen Leistungsgeschehen, Berlin.
9. IGES Institut für Gesundheits- und Sozialforschung (2006), Gesundheitswirtschaft Brandenburg – Stand und Entwicklung, Manuskript.
10. Berliner Senat (2006), Ressortübergreifende Steuerungsgruppe der Staatssekretäre für Wirtschaft, für Gesundheit und für Wissenschaft, Masterplan "Gesundheitsregion Berlin-Brandenburg".
11. Henke K-D, Mackenthun B, Schreyögg J (2004), The health care sector as economic driver: an economic analysis of the health care market in the city of Berlin, Journal of Public Health, 12: 339–345.
12. Kickbusch I (2006), Die Gesundheitsgesellschaft, Gamburg.
13. Neubauer G, Lewis P (2005), Gesundheit als Wirtschaftsfaktor im Untersuchungsraum München, München.

Chapter 5
Integrating Health in All Policies at the Local Level: Using Network Governance to Create 'Virtual Reorganization by Design'

Morton Warner and Nicholas Gould

Abstract The thesis of this chapter is that the Health in All Policy innovation process is only complete when national intentions have linked up with, and made a change to, 'practice' at the local level. Much is known about the way bureaucratic hierarchies attempt, but often fail, to make this happen, but much less so in relation to networks. For the latter, evidence is presented showing their superiority when policies are complex, requiring cross organizational action, and when the potential effort directed to their achievement is fragmented.

In the case of HiAP both situations apply. However, in the dialog between 26 of 32 countries meeting in Finland in 2006 to consider obstacles and driving forces in relation to HiAP, it is remarkable that no consideration is given to the possibility that the very nature of organizations, and what they represent to those who work in them, might be a root cause of the many years of relative failure to bring about multisectoral, interorganizational action.

Directed specifically toward improvement of interorganizational relationships, the chapter focuses on arrangements that can be put in place to overcome barriers to integrative action. These may be structural, procedural, financial, professional, or relate to status and legitimacy.

Ultimately, the aim is to achieve virtual reorganization, with the design of bringing together interorganizational effort to achieve health and social gain targets. This is Policy Innovation Number 1.

The journey to this end involves an understanding of what will:

- bring a diverse range of organizations to the table to form networks – using resources better, gaining wider skills, sharing risk and uncertainty, adaptive efficiencies, and legal or regulatory demands, and
- the crucial elements involved in network development if success is to be assured – the right choice of network type, relating to complexity of the

To the best of my knowledge none of the figures or boxes are protected by the copyright of others.

M.Warner (✉)
Welsh Institute for Health and Social Care, Glyntaff Campus, University of Glamorgan, Pontypridd, Wales
drmmwarner@tiscali.co.uk

problem, the specialist knowledge required, size, etc; an understanding of the organizational cultures of members; communication arrangements; and good governance.

This is Policy Innovation Number 2.

The chapter also introduces the 'neutral white space' concept – a zone between participating organizations where they can meet in an unfettered, less guarded way. Coordination of activity is key; and a particular role is described which involves 'attracting', 'guiding,' and brokering white space and virtual reorganizations' activities, that is working with networks in the space *and* assisting in mainstreaming the results of their creative thinking. This is Policy Innovation Number 3.

The evidential base which enabled the above approach to be developed was tested in an extensive 4-year action research project in South Wales, UK. This is reported here in case study form as a self-standing item at the end of the chapter. Policies which might provide a better quality of life and health for older people were developed through coordinated networks concerned with crime, transport, income and medication, and implemented by the partner organizations working in a virtually reorganized way.

Introduction

The thesis of this chapter is that the policy innovation process is only complete when high-level intentions have linked up with, and made a change to, 'practice'. The consequence, desirably, is improvement for the people, or of the situation, at which the policy is directed. This process we refer to as 'policy connect'. For this to happen not only must linkages be engineered *vertically* – and from 'bottom-up' as much as 'top-down' – but also *horizontally,* especially at the local level.

It is this horizontal axis which represents the crucial territory where new thinking is required which will recognize and aim to overcome the inertia and hostility often found within and between organizations which retards development. Usefully, Gareth Morgan [1], in his imaginative language of mental constraint, uses the expression 'psychic prisons', and suggests that members of organizations, and the actions they pursue, are constantly trapped by memories of the real or believed history.

Policy innovation, in the guise of calls for multisectoral action, is represented by the HiAP of the Council of the European Union [2]; and below is a summary of their considerations, and an invitation to the European Commission and Member States to act. What can be noted is that neither the preparatory meeting which preceded the Council's conclusions held in Finland [3], nor the conclusions themselves draw sufficient attention to the dynamics of interorganizational cooperation; but the former does have many other useful comments on the implementation of HiAP and these, too, are summarized below.

The second part of this chapter reviews the evidence on how in the practice of HiAP the interorganizational problems of multisectoral action might be overcome. This focuses on the use of well governed networks which operate in 'neutral' territory as a means of carrying forward the agenda at local level. The total span, from network activity directed at responding creatively to health targets, to the formation of virtual organizations charged with implementation, is referred to here as 'virtual reorganization by design' (VRD).

The third segment deals with the subject of 'coordination' and the role of coordinators, particularly as they are required to colonize the neutral territory, to cross organizational boundaries, and to broker action within the mainstream operations of participating bodies.

In the final section, an HiAP case study is presented – Project CHAIN (Community Health Alliances through Integrated Networks) – to illustrate how network theory was moved into practice and tested out in an action research programme activity in Wales, where the focus was on the broad-ranging needs of the elderly.

Health in All Policies

Both the WHO European Office in 1984 [4] and the Council of the European Union in 1991 [5] have put forward approaches committing their organizations to pursue multisectoral health policies. So, too, they have taken a concerted view that good health is influenced both by the actions of individuals and those of organizations.

In Health in All Policies in 2006 [3], the Union noted a range of health problems about which they had expressed concern between 2001 and 2006: alcohol-related harms (2001); stress and depression (2001); obesity (2001); healthy lifestyles – education, information, and communication (2003); alcohol and young people (2004); obesity, nutrition, and physical activity (2005); promotion of healthy lifestyles and prevention of Type 2 diabetes (2006); and women's health (2006). All, they observed, require a mixture of individual and multisectoral action if progress is to be made. And, they stressed that good health will be largely determined by matters beyond the purview of health care services.

Specifically, they welcomed (and endorsed, through invitation to Member States and the Commission to act) the thinking which came from a preparatory conference on Health in All Policies held in Kuopio, Finland, in September 2006, and which said:-

- Give greater consideration to health impacts in decision-making across policy sectors at different levels.
- Many policies with overlapping health objectives would benefit from intersectoral collaboration with common objectives.
- Public health and healthcare institutions and health professionals should act as advocates and experts for intersectoral work [6].

While there were other observations and actions proposed, those listed above are of the greatest relevance to the tasks set out for this chapter.

Of note, though, in a working paper [3] published from the conference a number of obstacles and driving forces for intersectoral action were identified following policy dialogs between 26 of the 32 countries participating.

Obstacles

Workload; inconsistencies between health and other sectors' objectives; health not having a very high priority in other sectors; the perception that only the Ministry of Health is responsible for health; and lack of evidence of what works and what does not.

Driving Forces

Incidental events (for example, in one country an accident initiated the alcohol strategy process); strong political leadership; scientific evidence; the presence of the theme on the EU agenda; shared values of health and well-being; awareness of health problems; public support; and personal contacts.

The content of these lists is, in most ways unremarkable, except that neither includes any consideration of the possibility that the very nature of organizations, and what they represent for those who work in them, might be a potential root cause of the many years of difficulty in bringing about multi-organizational, multisectoral coordinated action.

But, elsewhere in the same working paper, some explanation of the participants' thinking about the implementation and mechanisms that are supportive of cooperation is provided:

- Horizontal public health committees
- Formal consultations on, for example, legislation
- Ad hoc committees on specific initiatives
- Intersectoral policies and programmes
- Public health reporting (with the cooperation of other sectors)
- Formal communication between sectors (for example, bilateral meetings of permanent secretaries)
- EU coordination
- Health Impact Assessment
- Informal contacts

This list is heavily inclined toward action at national levels of policy; but elsewhere Ritsatakis and Järvisalo [7] give examples which range from local to international. Certainly in the 'local' HiAP case study with which this chapter concludes there are vestiges of a number of the mechanisms listed, although placed this time in the overall conceptual framework of 'virtual reorganization by design'.

Health in All Policies and the Determinants of Health – From Dahlgren and Whitehead to Modern Sweden

Dahlgren and Whitehead [8] as part of their work for the WHO European Office's, Health for All Programme, proposed the now famous sunrise diagram. Its naïve

Fig. 1 The determinants of health
Source [8]

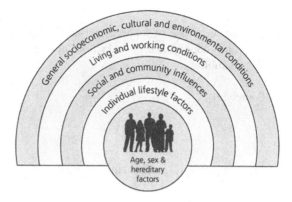

simplicity is worth repeating here (Fig. 1). But it is the underlying ramifications – the linking of political, economic, social, and biological components – which, for some time, made it difficult for the WHO to accept and embrace. Also, for us, starting with the 'what' of determinants is a far cry from addressing the essential of the arrangements that would require multisectoral and interorganizational cooperation – the 'how' – if the necessary synergies were to be achieved.

Twenty years later it is instructive to see what, if any, progress has been made in this regard. One example is Sweden's new public health strategy, published in 2003 [9], which is summarized by its objectives set out in Box 1. The first six are related to structural factors, the sort of things which can be molded by public opinion and political decision making at different levels. The last five concern lifestyle factors, which are under the influence of individuals, but where the social environment, too, plays an important part. In 2005 a Public Health Policy Report introduced 36 more detailed indicators and 47 subindicators to give greater specificity to the broad objectives.

Box 1: Swedish public health objectives

1. Participation and influence in society
2. Economic and Social Security
3. Secure and favorable conditions during childhood and adolescence
4. Healthier working life
5. Healthy and safe environments and products
6. Health and medical care that more actively promotes good health
7. Effective protection against communicable diseases
8. Safe sexuality and good reproductive health
9. Increased physical activity
10. Good eating habits and safe food

11. Reduced use of tobacco and alcohol, a society free from illicit drugs and doping and a reduction in the harmful effects of excessive gambling

Source [10]

More importantly, perhaps, the 2003 policy notes the following:

The 11 public health objectives involve an estimated 50 or so government agencies. In addition, municipalities and county councils have a major responsibility for conducting public health work on the local and regional levels, as it is on the local level that most of the decisions affecting people's actual living conditions are taken and the county councils have a responsibly to implement preventive measures under the Health and Medical Care Services Act. (p. 18)

It is to all those bodies ('the administration') that implementation is left, one early evaluation notes. "Governing with targets has its origins in the notion that administration possesses the best knowledge of how to implement measures. Accordingly the implementation process is completely delegated to the administration... governing with targets means telling the administration what to achieve but not what to do". [11]

Even then in Sweden, where the policy has been described as the first one representing "a third public health revolution" [12], few clues are given as to how implementation is to be executed. In part this is, no doubt, due to a reticence of the central government to move into the territory of other governmental levels, or the private sector. But also it recognizes the inherent issue that territory and power go hand in hand, and self-autonomy – often viewed as a sovereign right – will, if challenged, divert from the main intent of the exercise, improvements in public health.

Even by 2005 the Director for Public Health of the Ministry of Health and Social Affairs saw implementation involving "governmental directives to all concerned state agencies to take action on objectives under their sectoral responsibility" [13]. But Sweden is not alone in resorting to 'sectoral' calls and leaving multisectoral action, with its inevitable interorganizational stresses, to take care of itself. What does make it different, however, is the recognition, albeit in a cursory way, that target setting and implementation must be thought of in terms of political and organizational perspectives. In this they are more realistic than some other countries which have attempted to implement integration approaches more directly linked to clinical networks, with very little, or no recognition of the considerable need to address interorganizational relationships. Australia [14], England [15], and Scotland [16] are examples.

The Challenges to 'Local' Policy Innovation

Stakeholder Positions

Much of what is proposed later, in terms of essential processes to oil the wheels of interorganizational activity, is applicable to organizations working the policy to practice territories. But there are particular characteristics of 'local' situations which require specific consideration if the size and nature of the obstacles to be overcome are to be sufficiently understood. This is emphasized elsewhere in this volume by Sakellarides.

Hardy and his colleagues [17] have summarized the barriers underlying multi-sectoral cooperation, in terms of organizational integration problems, and these are set out in Fig. 2.

Of particular note is the inclusion (but at the end rather than at the outset) of organizational self interest and autonomy, competition for domains, and perceptions of the differential legitimacy of agencies with elected and appointed boards. It certainly must be remembered that at any local or regional level:-

- The range of organizations will be very wide, to include health services, local government, the voluntary and private sector, and citizens groups.
- Each organization will operate through separate strategies, with different management arrangements, and will likely employ a diverse range of professionals.

Addressing complex problems (such as the determinants of health) in a coordinated way across a large number of organizations (when there is a fragmentation of

Structural	– Fragmentation of service responsibilities across agency boundaries, within and between sectors – Competition-based systems of governance
Procedural	– Differences in planning horizons and cycles – Differences in budgetary cycles and procedures – Differences in information systems and protocols regarding confidentiality and access
Financial	– Differences in funding mechanisms and bases – Differences in stock and flows of financial resources
Professional	– Competing ideologies and values – Professional self-interest and autonomy and inter-professional competition for domains – Threats to job security – Conflicting views about clients/consumers interests and roles
Status & Legitimacy	– Organisational self-interest and autonomy and inter-organisational competition for domains – Differences in legitimacy between elected and appointed agencies

Fig. 2 Barriers to organisational integration

activity) requires innovative approaches, and here the evidence exists that 'network' formations are superior to hierarchical arrangements [18]. But what is the nature of the territory within which they might exist? It is important to identify this before proceeding with the discussion about network development *per se*.

The Need for Virtual Neutral Space

By choice, organizations will uphold their self-autonomous status and protect territory if a non-threatening alternative is not available. It is the mental construct of a neutral 'white space' at the outset of the change process that can provide an opportunity to overcome interorganization barriers. In the absence of such a neutral space, initiators of partnership arrangements have, in the past, often taken an approach aimed at breeching the thick defensive walls that surround organizations – only to see them built up as fast as they are knocked down by employees within.

The alternative way thinking has been summarized elsewhere:

> An organisational chart is depicted visually as a number of boxes, normally interconnected. The central area between the boxes indicates an absence of organisational activity, and this was titled as the neutral 'white space'. There are precedents for this idea: in network theory, one researcher, [19] has pioneered the concept of 'structural holes', which both impose constraints and offer opportunities. In this new territory, untrammelled by organisational pre-conditions and assumptions, creative network activity can take place which results in the redesign of services [20].

Network activities are sustained through governance arrangements which involve social mechanisms such as trust, commitment, and the threat of exclusion from the network [19]. But even though governance suggests a means of regulating activity in the white space, for practical purposes we are forced back to the problem of 'who' or 'what' is to be responsible for coordination.

To go further, the construction of such a design, where organizations are located around the virtual 'white space', creates both 'borders' and 'boundaries'. And it is Paul Tillich, the 20th century theologian, who has observed that 'the border line is the truly propitious place for acquiring knowledge' [21], and 'Boundaries are as windows and doors, not prison walls' [22]. Agreement by organizations to position themselves around the space (or accept that they are already so positioned) is an important first step to becoming engaged in the formation of networks to problem-solve across the organizational boundaries. For those with responsibility for implementing HiAP it is important that they initiate discussions around this agenda item very early on.

Network development aspects are dealt with at some length in the following section; and the coordination of network activity and the link to mainstream organizational operations will come after this, and is illustrated by the case study.

Network Development

Given an almost intrinsic requirement for HiAP intentions to be implemented through networks, and the key part that networks can play in policy innovation, it is useful to have some grounding in the important literature that exists on their formation and characteristics.

In the early 1980s, Aldrich and Whetten [23] commented in the "Handbook of Organizational Design" that the network concept is used generally as a metaphor. Nearly 20 years later, working in the human services field, Milward and Provan [24] made a similar remark. 'Networks' tends to remain a vague notion despite their long-standing recognition as a distinct form providing a clear alternative *modus operandi* to markets and to bureaucratic hierarchies [25]. Given the perception of their increasing importance in achieving integrated action, networks require a richer and more detailed description if their full potential is to be realized.

Here the aim is to provide a conceptual core that is usable for interorganizational network design and management in support of HiAP. Knowledge gained from decades of empirical and theoretical research has reached the stage where network development can be approached scientifically. The conditions necessary for network formation and for subsequent structure and governance are now accepted by theorists, and are linked within an environmental context that also includes culture and technology. In practice much network development is intuitive, and often misses out on employing key success factors.

Network Formation and Emergence

(What conditions are favorable to the formation of interorganizational networks?)

Responses to the question centre on both global and local activity. The global context continues to be one of rapid change, whether technological, political, or social; and this has resulted in challenges to the dominance of the more routenized, 'Fordist' methods of organization.

Investigating the local conditions favorable to the emergence of network organization has also attracted considerable research [26]. In this respect, Grandori and Soda [27] review cases in the context of their paradigmatic reference frames – for example, the need for legitimacy within an institutional framework and used here in the discussion that follows Fig. 2. Ebers [28], in developing this theme, employs the notion of organizational ecology and gives prominence to Oliver's work on the determinants of interorganizational relationships [29].

Derived from these and other reviews, Fig. 3 presents a composite of the primary conditions for network formation.

Applying the factors to intersectoral action, they can be grouped under three conventional headings or reference frames:

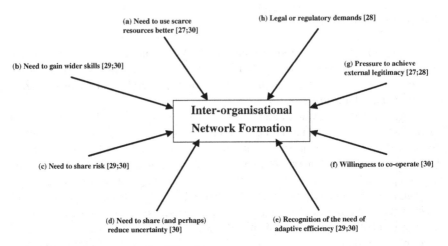

Fig. 3 Factors influencing network formation

- *Resources* (a and b) – In isolation, sectors and organizations often duplicate some services whilst being unable to resource others. Furthermore, they may lack specific expertise and need to interface with other organizations, who in turn often have inadequate financial resources. Networks, then, can be given cause to form when resources are scarce or used inefficiently.
- *Contingencies* (c to f) – Human service organizations often serve populations where large numbers of clients and communities suffer from multiple problems and their requirements continuously change. In this situation, characterized by high risk and uncertainty and requiring adaptive efficiency, network structures may emerge. These external stimuli may exist alongside an already present willingness for interagency cooperation.
- *Institutional* (g and h) – Networks in themselves may be perceived as a more democratic and, in the current milieu, a more legitimate form of organizing than hierarchies. Prospective network members may also feel that they can derive greater legitimacy in the external world by being seen to be part of a larger grouping. It may also be that governments regulate activity in favor of networks by financing not-for-profit organizations to assist in the delivery of integrated action, or by relaxing rules about the pooling of public funds to encourage partnerships.

In isolation or in combination the factors represent necessary pre-conditions not just for network formation but also joint ventures, partnerships and alliances [30], and Box 2 provides a description of the differences between networks and partnerships' two terms which are often interchanged and can lead to confusion.

If 'willingness to cooperate' is lacking, even the presence of seven of the eight factors may not be sufficient to guarantee network formation. Furthermore, when the network form offers organizational advantages, *effort* may still be required to overcome structural inertia or the other reasons for potential network failure [31, 32]. Reference to 'effort' serves as a reminder that networks require management as a professional activity recognized in its own right [33]. A detailed case study of 'health gain' developments in Wales shows how hard this is [34]. The common agenda brought about a wide willingness to cooperate, but considerable and concerted activity was involved in managing the process of advancement.

Box 2: Partnerships and networks – What is the difference?

Both partnerships and networks use contracts to contain or direct people's behavior. That is, a contract is a form of 'governance'.

Traditional partnerships may be completely governed by contract. But it is difficult to see a large network being governed by a single legal contract – multiple legal contracts, maybe, but even this is begins to strain accepted definitions of 'organizational network'.

So, in summary:

- All partnerships can be considered as networks. But the reverse is not true.
- Partnerships can be thought of as special sorts of networks.
- Networks and Partnerships are both entities. We can point to actual examples in the world.
- Networks and Modern Partnerships share a common approach to organization in that they rely on trust, commitment and mutual respect (social contract).
- Traditional Partnerships have their basis in a legal contract.
- Ideally, networks have their basis in social contracts.
- Partnerships have a small number of people or organizations at their core.
- A network may involve dozens of organizations.
- Networks have a distinctive form of analysis. This can be used to study partnerships.
- Partnerships do not have a distinctive form of analysis.

The younger generations might, at one level, have less difficulty in participating in networks in the future – the easy availability and cheapness of a new range of telecommunication mechanisms has ensured this. And with chat rooms and MySpace, they construct their own white space in an organic way, and are influenced to form networks motivated by many of the same factors as their organizational cousins. This presents major possibilities in the field of public health, itself intrinsically a network activity.

Network Structures

(What types of network are there?)

People are largely familiar with 'networking' both at work and in less formal situations. In this context a network of primary school friends, for example, can be represented graphically by a set of dots (the friends) joined by lines (the presence of friendship). In this case the 'sociogram' [35] may vary almost daily. However, the underlying pattern or form will probably remain constant. Grandori and Soda [27] ask: "Can we develop a classification of network forms that might be conducive to a comparison among them?" If so, we would then be able to consider the difference in *structure* between, say, a community-based health advocacy alliance and a homecare delivery network [36, 37]. This would be helpful in making the right choice of network type for each of the wide variety of HiAP challenges.

It is in this respect the contribution of Hage and Alter [38] in developing two typological formats warrants particular attention given their extensive analysis of health and social care networks. In the first, drawing on numerous case studies, they present a *descriptive* typology of interorganizational relationships and networks. Then, utilizing findings from their own research on health and social care service delivery systems, they generate a more *technical classification* of network structure.

The Descriptive Typology

Central to this are the notions of obligation, promotion, and production, items which correspond with progressively higher levels of complexity. Obligation is mainly related to the presence of exchange in social networks, and simple coordination suffices in limited complexity situations. Promotion involves greater formality, for instance to coordinate robust communications. Development and production networks have their own specific complex requirements which require a high degree of cooperation and coordination. As a response to Grandori and Soda's challenge concerning the classification of network forms, the Alter-Hage descriptive typology is helpful.

The Technical Classification

Continuing then, Alter and Hage conjecture there are only four basic types of networks. Recently, this has received partial confirmation by groups of US researchers working in the health field [39, 40]. Using the dimensions of differentiation, centralization, and integration (in contrast to complexity), they also identified four network formats. However, network size was not a dimension of their analysis.

The inclusion in Fig. 4 of both complexity *and* differentiation requires comment. To be concise, reflecting on the nature of integrated interorganizational action

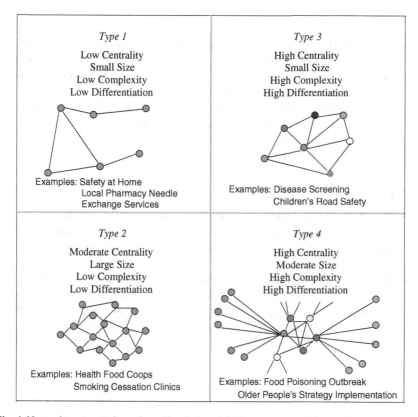

Fig. 4 Networks: structural typology (developed after Hage and Alter, [41])

suggests that 'complexity' alone does not adequately convey the full variation in activity – hence the inclusion in the foregoing discussions and in Fig. 4 of 'differentiation' – the span of the knowledge base provided by the participants – so as to provide descriptive power.

While the total number of network types needs further research, current evidence suggests it is probably countable on the fingers of one hand. This small number, Alter and Hage suggest, may result from evolutionary processes related to the global technical drivers considered earlier and their impact on the emergence, formation and management of networks. Furthermore, unfocussed management may produce inappropriate designs that are difficult to sustain within the natural ecology of network development (see, for example, Hannan and Freeman [42]).

In the above figure examples are cited for each of the network types. Often the network design chosen 'on the ground' comes about somewhat accidentally; but conscious and more considered decision-making about the type of network to be employed should lead to higher levels of success in implementation. In summary, the characteristics of each example are as follows:

Type 1

- **Safety at Home,** designed to prevent accidents and injuries, mostly to older people. Includes securing carpets, testing electric blankets and heating, and installing smoke alarms. Carried out by groups of volunteers and their friends with minimum training.
- **Local Pharmacy Needle Exchange Services**, designed to control infectious diseases among drug users. Local pharmacies group together to obtain supplies, exchange intelligence and further extend the service as part of a broader Type 2 public health network.

Type 2

- **Health Food Cooperatives,** made up of local people buying in bulk, with nutritional consideration of importance. The large size is required for economic visibility, but the concept is simple and the range of knowledge required is limited.
- **Smoking Cessation Clinics,** consisting of a large number of linked local venues serving those who have decided to quit. Provide advice, support and nicotine patches through volunteers and generally nonprofessional staff, though organized by professional staff. The density of clinics locally is a characteristic of their success.

Type 3

- **Disease Screening,** where the aim is to spot susceptibility to disease. Many schemes function around a centralized call/recall system, together with a linked network, ranging from laboratories or other diagnostic services to primary care and medical consultants, each employing highly differentiated knowledge.
- **Children's Road Safety,** which involves inputs from a wide range of organizations and where the police and hospital accident and emergency departments occupy the hub of the network. Other highly differentiated local stakeholders might include: local authority road and engineering departments, and schools and parents.

Type 4

- **A Food Poisoning Outbreak,** where the core network is configured from a number of highly differentiated multidisciplinary agencies, which might include the public health service, the centre for disease control environment, health, and the police. Beyond them are hospital and primary care practitioners providing treatment services, and trading standards as required.
- **Older People's Strategy Implementation,** which at local levels may involve a care network including health, social services, leisure services, education, employer organizations and financial advisors, all contributing

to the concept of active citizenship. Each organization may increase its geographic coverage and equitability of access through expanded linkages.

Not only can it be seen that the choice of appropriate network type is important, but it may also be inferred that individual networks may need to undergo a transition to another form as the range of tasks change. In either case, there is a specialist coordination, design, and monitoring function to be exercised by those with specific responsibility for network development.

Network Governance

(How is purposeful activity generated and maintained in a network?)

Essentially, the answer here relates to matters of coordination and control, that is governance [43]. The more common experience of hierarchies and market settings, where the role of authority and price mechanisms are obvious, leads to concerns about the perceived vagueness of the corresponding mechanisms of coordination and control which are applied to networks [44]. For example, in a network for which one role might be the monitoring of substance abuse, how do care workers and law enforcers interact in the absence of common line management? Of course, such issues go to the heart of the 'integration' challenge wherein the division of labor needs to be reconnected in a coherent manner [45].

There are, of course, a range of coordination and control mechanisms that networks share with other organizational forms. Grandori and Soda [27] include incentive arrangements and information systems as well as the planning and control-by-results. Networks also rely heavily on a good communications infrastructure and the availability of personnel with highly tuned negotiation skills: together, these reflect the enhanced role of so-called 'social mechanisms' in maintaining activity. One description of network governance is that it:

> involves a select, persistent, and structured set of autonomous firms (or nonprofit agencies) engaged in creating products or services based on implicit and open-ended contracts to adapt to environmental contingencies and to co-ordinate and safeguard exchanges. These contracts are socially – not legally – binding [18].

The authors expand on the social dimensions, in terms of restricted access, macroculture, collective sanctions and reputation, but others also give prominence to trust and commitment [1, 46].

Selection for network membership is attained through a recognition that competency exists which will complement or supplement network goals (see, for example, [47]). For day-to-day management of integrated care networks recognition of the primacy of the social mechanisms of governance is important. Sustaining network activity depends on mutual encouragement of trust and commitment, whilst not forgetting the consequences of malfeasance. In many ways, it is all threats and promises – or sticks and carrots [48].

Constructing the Network Design

(What is the minimum set of concepts for a useful representation of network activity?)

Linking the Components

It is necessary at this stage to link the network components thus far described – relating to structure and governance – to the often-changing elements of 'culture' and 'technology'. Also, to move us from metaphor requires availability of accurate descriptive models. In this respect, "Leavitt's Diamond" [49] proves useful; it represents organizational arrangements using four dimensions: social structure, technology, participants and goals. In Fig. 5 we retain Leavitt's (social) structure and technology but replace 'goals ' with 'culture' and 'participants' by 'governance'.

The notion of organizational culture includes goals, thus a gain in descriptive power. The use of governance is seen as more appropriate for network organizations because it is more dynamic, implying not just the involvement of participants but also their social interactions and relationships, including the role of leadership.

Other authors have also made modifications to Leavitt which we have adopted. Scott [50] set the four dimensions within an external environment, here referred to as 'global'. Smith et al. [51], Homburg et al. [52], and their colleagues developed

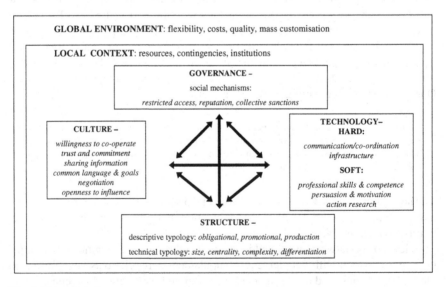

Fig. 5 Network design

the tradition of also giving emphasis to the need to adapt the dimension within a local context.

Throughout (as indicated by the two-headed arrows), the *interdependence* of dimensions within each given environment is stressed. Looking at the dimensions in this way offers further network insights.

To have a more complete understanding of the role of networks within intersectoral action, or more importantly how to promote a highly integrated approach, involves further consideration of the technology and culture elements in the figure and the interactions between them, as well as with structure and governance.

It is important to recall that integrating multiorganizational activity involves many technologies and tasks that need to complement and reinforce each other. These are made up of the skills and competencies of practitioners; and the concern or bringing together through appropriate communication and coordination at all levels, from strategic planning through to practice. In this respect, information systems can form a dual function of providing valuable intelligence to individual practitioners as well as recording patterns of service or programme delivery which, in turn, will assist overall coordination. The development of powerful computer-supported information technologies has transformed the tasks associated with both communication and coordination; and the growth of networks owes much to these far-reaching developments, including the knowledge exchange potential of the Internet. In the broadest sense, networks in totality can be considered as information value chains – as knowledge is generated, it is circulated. Hernández-Aguado has, elsewhere in this volume, developed this theme as a major exposition.

The possibilities associated with 'hard' technologies, such as teleconferencing and the Internet can, in themselves, encourage the development of virtual teams [53]. The further integration of activities, using virtual means, represents an extension of the networked teams and networks of team that have been a longstanding feature of the organization of community care [54]. However, the 'soft' technologies of influence, persuasion and motivation are crucial to generating trust and commitment on the part of clinical and public health practitioners: the trend toward virtuality needs to be balanced with the need to maintain face-to-face relationships [55].

As to culture, a 'willingness to cooperate' as a network pre-condition continues to be a key core value and norm of desired behavior [56]. In addition, a collaborative ethos can lead to a better convergence of expectations and goals, for instance through recognizing the need for sharing information for the benefit of patients, clients or communities.

To overcome the interorganizational constraints posed by the use of professional jargon, the development of a common language within integrated action is important [57]. Notwithstanding the possibilities for increased on cooperation, networks can also be prone to destructive competition and conflict just like hierarchies and markets [58]. However, in attempting to balance tensions and conflicts of interest, networks more naturally reconcile power differentials through the elevation of mutual influence and negotiation [59].

Virtual Coordination

We move now from the 'what' of networks to 'how' they should be managed in order to achieve efficient integrated interorganizational action, a key platform of the multisectoral approach of HiAP. Management of coordination is a further element of the policy innovation process.

The Integration Challenge

Theoretically, any debate about the nature and form of integration can be interpreted in terms of the 'Coasian' question. Coase asked, "Why doesn't all industrial activity take place within one large organization?" [60]. Less directly, Lawrence and Lorsch's [61] concern with both differentiation and integration raised the same fundamental issue from the viewpoint of contingency theory, and suggest there is no universal blueprint for organization. Alter and Hage [41] adapted this approach for their investigation of *'organizations working together'* through a study of fifteen different health and welfare networks. This research should also cause us to consider carefully any strategy of 'integration-by-barrier-removal'. For example, formal combination of service provision for some aspects of elder care may well be advantageous for all parties. But there are clear limits. Cases of elder abuse do not justify the incorporation of the police into a care organization. Coase's question raises an important point about 'total integration'.

Barriers to integration have a parallel in the concept of 'boundaries'. Tillich [22] describes various types of social, theological and physical boundaries as fundamental to the human psyche. Some psychoanalytic traditions emphasize boundary and space [62]. In the organizational literature, boundaries are a familiar term [63–65]. During the 1970s, Aldrich and others developed the notion of 'boundary spanning role' in the interorganizational field [23, 66, 67]. With the recent growth of interest in partnerships, alliances and networks, there has been renewed interest in this notion.

Briefly contrasting and comparing barriers and boundaries is instructive. As a metaphor, a barrier connotes the impenetrable, something resisting access or change. In institutional settings, barriers may well be appropriate as a means of guarding rights and defining responsibilities. Human services often fall into this category. On the other hand, when considering issues such as user-involvement or the limits of total integration, boundary is a more useful term. Boundaries can be elastic or permeable offering the possibility of adjustment or diffusion and exchange. In achieving integration by means other than formal combination, 'spanning boundaries' replaces 'removing barriers'. The question now arises as to who or what does this boundary spanning.

Boundary Spanning and Virtual Coordination

In positing the boundary spanning role, Aldrich [23, 67] investigated both boundary personnel and linking-pin organizations. No mutual exclusivity is implied.

Linking-pin organizations may well contain boundary personnel, though not necessarily in the Internet era. Williams has taken forward research on individual 'boundary spanners'. He identifies four emerging competency areas:

- *Building and Sustaining Relationships* – dimensioned by: communicating and listening / understanding and conflict resolution / personal character / and trust.
- *Managing within Nonhierarchical Domains* – dimensioned by: influencing / negotiating / brokering / and networking.
- *Managing Interdependencies* – no dimensions are specified.
- *Managing Roles and Accountabilities* – no dimensions specified. [68, 69]

These competency areas were generated by a qualitative method. There may well be a degree of redundancy, for example between 'communicating and listening' and 'negotiating'. Further, all the management areas probably can be subsumed under the one heading 'Managing within Nonhierarchical Domains'. We also note that data was gathered from individuals employed as boundary spanners within existing agencies. This positional restriction of the role is potentially problematic. Aldrich and Whetten [23] record that "It follows that boundary spanners in richly joined organizations would experience more role conflict as they attempt to cope with the conflicting experiences of internal and external reference groups". That is, there appear to be inherent limitations on boundary spanners sited within existing organizations. Despite these shortcomings, Williams has provided researchers and practitioners with the means of thinking more precisely about boundary spanning personnel.

As for linking-pin organizations, Aldrich and Whetten write:

Linking-pin organizations that have extensive and overlapping ties to different parts of a network play the key role in integrating a population of organizations. Having ties to more than one action-set or subsystem, linking-pin organizations are the nodes through which a network is loosely joined. [23]

There exist a number of similar conceptions. Within the systems paradigm, Trist suggested that the 'referent organization' is one that "...would not be an operating agency but would perform a regulative and developmental function." [70]. Trist qualifies the regulative function by insisting on the need for self-regulation in democratic domains where the recognition of interdependence is understood as central. Balancing third-party regulation and self- regulation is an evolutionary process taking the form of the *'negotiated order'*. This comment points to a fundamental tension in the development of networks, especially in human services. The self-organizing advantages of networks often have to be tempered by organizational and professional accountabilities. By negotiated order, Trist indicates that it is likely that interorganizational collaborations will require extended dialogs and purposeful actions in order to achieve beneficial outcomes and outputs. Other similar conceptions include: the imaginary organization leader [59], the strategic centre [71], and the network administrative organization [72]. All these organizational innovations transcend the original boundary spanning notion in one fundamental way. In contrast to the boundary spanners studied by Williams [68], these referent organizations are autonomous from their served population. This observation points to a stronger version of the boundary spanning role which requires linkage through both communication and coordination.

Reference back to the complexities inherent in the implementation of the Swedish Public Health Objectives (Box 2) quickly bring the above considerations into perspective. For HiAP to be successful the tensions about organizational autonomy that will be ongoing, in spite of networked activity, need managing at a variety of coordinative nodes and also across the nodal points.

The following features early in the text of *Multiskilling: Health Unit Coordination for the Health Care Provider*:

> Financial coordination: arrangement of methods to allow payment for services provided by the facility; includes working closely with insurance carriers, government programs, and personal payment programs. [73]

This is a reminder both of the requirement for coordination in respect of the barriers to integration and that health care providers have multiple links beyond their organizational boundaries. In their seminal work, *Organizations,* March and Simon state [74], "The problem of arranging the signalling system for interdependent conditional activities is the coordination problem." Such a definition is consistent with a rational systems approach to organization based on the behavioral sciences [50]. There is a mechanical and automated character to the definition that accords with the above statement of financial coordination. By contrast, consider:

> Coordination is also described as **the quality of the relationship** between human actors in a working system and is **often** equated with co-operation. [41]

'*Quality of the relationship*' is a broad term that could include technical communications issues. It is perhaps more suggestive of the extent of trust, respect, commitment, shared goals and values and other 'soft' aspects of human interactions that coalesce to produce cooperation. The inclusion of '*often*' implies a conflation of cooperation and coordination that is not altogether correct. Not only does cooperation require coordination but so do conflict and competition [58]. There is an implication that coordination is essentially neutral and we make qualifications, for example, by referring to cooperative coordination as distinct from the competitive coordination in a market.

Hage and Alter [38] conclude that coordination is a process that in cooperative settings culminates in integration. Following Thompson [75], they also indicate that integration depends on the process of coordination at different organizational levels. Administrative coordination may take the form of formal contracts. Operational task coordination of patient/client flow has its own distinctive characteristics. These different 'horizontal' coordination formats need to be aligned 'vertically'; that is, further coordination. In the public sector, there are at least six vertical levels in the policy to service delivery chain: legislators, civil servants, chief executive officers, managers, practitioners and the general public. If we also take into consideration that "... the very proliferation of services constrains the service providers from functioning as a coordinated system" [76], then the coordination problem begins to take on a daunting scale.

Thinking more positively, the above analysis does offer an approach to the coordination jungle that may in turn lead to paths through it. Malone and Crowston's interdisciplinary study of coordination offers precise guidance:

> If coordination is defined as **managing** (inter-) **dependencies,** then further progress should be possible by **characterizing different kinds of** (inter-) **dependencies and identifying the coordination processes that can be used to manage them.** [77]

By inserting the parentheses into this definition, we have brought it into line with the standard interorganizational terminology (cf. Williams above: "managing interdependencies"). The definition is useful in two ways. First, and universally, it provides a clear focus on the technical aspects of coordination: characterizing (inter-) dependencies and then identifying processes. Second, and particularly, it offers a precise approach to the central challenge of integrated action. Malone and Crowston's first step in the coordination process – characterizing different kinds of (inter-) dependencies – necessarily implies the complementary process of characterizing *independencies*. Given that the barriers to integration could be thought of as arising from *independencies* and, as discussed above, barriers may be re-interpreted as boundaries, then we can begin to think more creatively about integration in this three step process. The first characterize dependencies, interdependencies, and independencies. The second re-interpret these characterizations in terms of barriers (forming types of inviolable autonomy) and boundaries (enclosing negotiable zones). And the third identifies the appropriate coordination processes that preserve barriers, re-form boundaries and ultimately generate integration.

In Summary:

- Not all integrated action formats can be achieved by removing the barriers to integration.
- We need to think both in terms of barriers and boundaries.
- Integration can be mediated by boundary spanners or linking-pin organizations.
- Stronger versions of the boundary spanning role emphasize both communication and coordination.
- Coordination involves understanding the range of dependencies and designing appropriate processes that result in integration.

Conclusions

The application of network governance will not be easy in the HiAP approach. Despite a new wide-scale growth of the network form, misgivings have been expressed about their application in the human service activities that might represent HiAP at the local level, where traditionally hierarchies have been the norm. Understandably, particular questions arise about accountability and leadership. In many ways, networks require a change of mindset. For example, instead of "Who is responsible?" we need to ask "Who or what is responsible?" Individuals may have defined coordination roles, but it is the network as a whole that is ultimately responsible.

The earlier definition of network governance stressed social rather than legally binding contracts – formal contracts are generally seen as being hierarchical in nature, and their introduction, it is claimed by some, would contaminate network purity [78]. The leadership qualities required in both hierarchies and networks have much in common. But it is the need to work primarily through social and other obligational approaches, as a cuckoo in many organizational nests that places special requirements on network leaders, or virtual organization coordinators.

The literature on multiorganizational partnerships and networks is substantial and broad, both in terms of the criteria necessary for their successful development, and in providing evaluations of such arrangements. Indeed, an international group convenes annually on a global basis to further the approaches in a wide range of subject areas [79].

The starting point for local change, along the lines required in HiAP, is for there to be a shift of emphasis on 'inputs' and 'outputs' to one that is guided strategically by the notion of 'investment' and 'outcomes'. "Let the idea be in charge", seems to be a theme emerging in Sakellarides' chapter; and this is that health and social gain for individuals and communities must form the central plank of all multisectoral activity. Through inclusive partnerships, all stakeholders can contribute to network activity; and the initial consideration of health and social targets and target setting is an important activity that gives networks a sense of purpose and alignment with personal values. Local competition and cooperation can be seen as synergistic once personal relationships have a basis of understanding.

The setting of specific but broad-ranging health and social gain targets jointly by two or more agencies also serves important purposes:

- First, targets if set properly provide the network with a sense that it is possible to follow a particular strategic direction and contribute to the achievement of policy goals, ensuring policy connects to practice [80].
- Second, the *process* involved in face-to-face target setting is central to the generation of trust, respect and commitment between individuals and agencies [81].

Additionally, during this process, 'partners at the dance' should emerge, to use Kaluzny's apt term [36]. Further, and to continue the analogy, agencies will swap the lead depending on the problems being addressed; and different virtual organizations will be constructed to solve particular problems, each with their own leader.

That networks can be responsive to a variety of influences is part of their attraction, and can result in interesting organizational hybrids [78]. This is reason enough for better conceptualization and a considered use of the design dimensions. Without a sound knowledge of networks, a series of misplaced or ill-timed interventions may result in inefficiency and ineffectiveness of network activity or outright network failure. Facilitation of links between HiAP implementation groups and local members of MOPAN (Multi-Organizational Partnerships, Alliances and Networks) would be advantageous in this regard [79]. The case study at the end of the chapter serves to illustrate the approaches used to employ the design dimensions and to overcome potential dysfunctional activity.

Overall, what the process of local implementation of HiAP requires is good management and coordination, and the introduction of governance mechanisms which are both 'loose' and 'tight'. A cadre of senior people with the necessary preparation to perform as 'coordinators' along the lines described earlier will be required: and this role varies considerably from that of a line manager, both in terms of the need for constant repositioning, and accountability.

Finally, there comes the need to accept that multisectoral arrangements are inherently messy and that networked activity across organizations needs governance. The current fragmentation of effort with which we are familiar comes about not by accident but because it is easier to manage 'within' rather than 'across' organizations. The result may be a dislocation that is convenient to live with. But it must be accepted, albeit slowly, that the complexity of the multisectoral action required to improve the determinants of health requires alternative approaches beyond those possible through hierarchical silo-bound activities. Networks well governed, and organizations virtually reorganized across sectors, are a challenge to policy innovators, but ones that it is necessary to meet head on.

A Health in All Policies Case Study at the Local Level: Project CHAIN (Community Health Alliances Through Integrated Networks)

Project Setting and Background

The formation of community alliances and networks over the period from 2000 to 2004 came from a multisectoral partnership of: the Welsh Assembly Government; a county borough council; a local health commissioning group; two NHS provider trusts; voluntary sector organizations; and a university institute. The partnership aimed to investigate the potential of virtual reorganization by design (VRD) as a contribution to improving the quality of life of older people living within the council's boundaries. In keeping with the action research base of the project, specific objectives emerged through a managed process which is described below.

The County Borough of Rhondda Cynon Taf (population 240,000) was formerly at the heart of coal mining in South Wales. The post-industrial legacy of that era presents a challenge to public health agencies. The area ranks as one of the most deprived in Europe, with standardized mortality well below average and a particularly high incidence of cardiovascular and respiratory disease. Meeting the present health deficits through quality health care, while simultaneously addressing the determinants of health to be tackled by health promotion and public health measures, offered a considerable challenge to the efforts of all agencies and for CHAIN. Moreover, the industrial legacy is not restricted to health deficits. The people of the Borough reside typically in villages originally based around the now defunct mines. The relative independence of these communities is deepened by their location in series of valleys, some of which are dead-end. Planning health and social care facilities is problematic, and further exacerbated by difficulties in the transportation infrastructure. A detailed knowledge of how these factors interact was important in terms of network building.

The Concept

The central policy innovation behind CHAIN, the need for VRD, stemmed from the following observations:

> "Whilst reorganisation implies change, most often what is proposed is incremental in nature; and though it might raise the potential for conflict it can be accommodated by organisations or professional groups which have to consider it using their existing structures and committees. Structural conflict is OK! It allows for mutual recrimination followed by collective admiration. Re-design, however, is more fundamental in what it attempts to do; and with its potential for moulding the future, challenges the existing structures, which are most often based on historical precedents. It causes frictional conflict by crossing previously well-defined boundaries, and takes both proponents and opponents of an innovative idea into new, more risky, territory.

> Reorganisation when applied to the public sector is accorded a variety of positive-sounding metaphors: it is challenged, efficient and integrational, bringing about greater choice and seamlessness of care or service. This is attractive language for the politician focussing on a three year window of opportunity for change.

> Re-design, whenever it is contemplated, is likened to a tidal wave, the result of which is likely to be chaos". [82]

CHAIN is a working example of VRD which aims to implement organizational change without the usual traumas and distractions. Figure 6 displays the elements of VRD in an intersectoral setting and represents a template for integrative activities

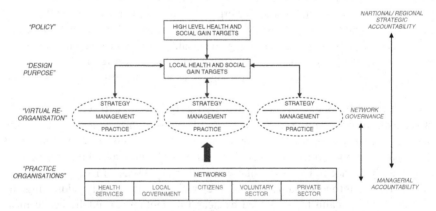

Fig. 6 Virtual reorganization by design to improve the publics' health: The structural elements
Source [85]

[83, 84]. Notable is the leading and guiding role played by the setting of high level and local targets [84].

The design orientations and components inherent to VRD in this model are those it set out earlier in the chapter.

Development Processes

Defining the Cast of Stakeholders

This was an important activity and took place against a background that managers tended to favor incremental involvement, *at the appropriate time*. In CHAIN, decisions were taken to maximize involvement from the outset, whilst recognizing that some staging of phases would be an essential component of a development process.

In broad terms the three phases that took place and the stakeholders were as follows:

Initiation and Mapping

- A Project Board, made up of representatives of the funding partners, gave the project legitimacy and a mandate to "contributing to older people's quality of life".
- Three Older People's Forums (constructed under a national programme of Better Government for Older People) were consulted, and their own quality of life consultations incorporated into the agenda.
- A Strategy and Policy Integration Group (SPIG), formed by senior managers, often deputy chief executives, and drawn from all the partnering organizations and the voluntary sector, were responsible for detailed agenda setting and commissioning of networks.

The SPIG took on the role of assuring horizontal integration. Initially, it performed two main tasks. First, it began the process of identifying specific health and social gain target areas that would ultimately generate objectives to underpin the quality of life aim. Second, it analysed the strategic documents of the partners to answer the question: "At the policy level, how joined up are we in relation to the quality of life aspirations of older people?" In a nutshell, the answer came back: "Not very integrated at all."

Broadening

Middle managers and practitioners from across all agencies responded in detail to the target areas identified by the SPIG. Increasing awareness of CHAIN made possible recruitment to integrated management and practitioners groups. Their members, together with participants from other agencies also identified at this time, were vital to the activities of the networks which later were to operate in the white space.

Consolidation

The findings of the analysis of current levels of collaboration were presented to two open conferences. Two questions were of crucial interest in respect of the work: Did it

- provide a reasonable picture or map of the local care system?
- contain the basis for action in relation to the older people's quality of life priorities?

Both were answered in the affirmative, and the conferences were characterized by a high degree of support and promises of commitment.

The Proposed Integrated Network Activity

Putting together the various data, information and knowledge gained from all the stakeholders, many issues had emerged for consideration by the SPIG, which was charged with reducing these to a workable number for proposed network activity. The selection criteria were:

- consistency with the older people's quality of life priorities;
- keep in line with the researched views gathered from service providers and commissioners;
- benchmarkable in respect of the National Service Framework for Older People and other public sector publications, policy drives and legislated procedures – particularly those issued by the Welsh Assembly Government;
- feasibility in respect of existing resources and the history of joint-working, with the additional criterion that the issues should be challenging though with a good chance of positive outcomes;
- that issues be cross-cutting, in a way that would in themselves require collaborative activities (that is: people could not retreat into their 'boxes').

Figure 7, below, indicates the networks that represented the range of CHAIN's activity, and in themselves they formed a second policy innovation.

The following short description sketches the raison d'être of the networks:-

Income Improvement

This network was established given the absolute priority accorded to the problem by local older people. The core involves a large range of interests. Prominent are older people themselves and representatives from the Carers' Support Project. Amongst providers from the statutory sector, the Department of Work and Pensions notably are working alongside colleagues from NHS Trusts. Two interrelated subnetworks addressed two strands of this issue:

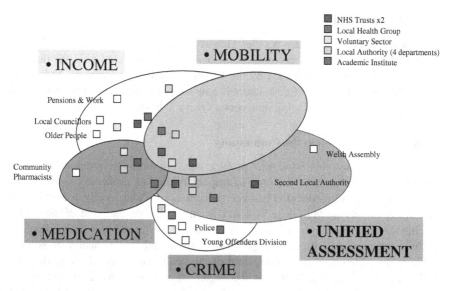

Fig. 7 'CHAIN' issue-based networks – Health in All Policies Source [86]

- Building on the successful Better Government for Older People initiative in which improved take up of benefits was encouraged, the first concentrated on further increasing that awareness by leveraging existing information resource points, e.g. libraries.
- The second principally targeted at the unnecessary draw-down that statutory bodies make on the limited incomes of older people, for example, the cumulative car parking fees paid by a husband visiting his wife confined to hospital by a fractured neck of femur.

Reducing the Fear of Crime

Contacts with the Older People's Forums confirmed this issue as seriously undermining peace of mind and general well-being in spite of crime figures reducing. This is a wide-ranging network of agencies and also involves the Police and the Media. Results are encouraging, with fear of crime reporting a reduction.

Mobility

Considering the 'support for independence' aim of the project, mobility both within the home and the wider community was chosen as an enveloping item, that is, it would offer the opportunity of very wide network development. For example, work included both the setting up of a post-discharge community reablement team as well as a review of local transport arrangements by the local authority to support general social activities.

Unified Assessment

Not an issue raised by older people! However, given that assessment underpins access to a large range of services, its inclusion was considered vital for integration. It was later to be mandated by the Welsh Assembly Government. Still in its relative infancy, this form of assessment is now seen as a requirement for integrated action, for example, in reducing unnecessary stays in hospital.

Managing Medication in the Community

In terms of history, this issue was problematic. For instance, previous attempts to resolve the problem of the precise responsibilities of homecare assistants in the administering of medication had been acrimonious. Additionally, a community pharmacist supplying Multidose System Dispensers was on the point of withdrawing the service due to overuse and lack of funding: this action was deemed potentially to put hundreds of older people at risk. By attempting to customize service delivery the pharmacist was falling foul of the health authority's lack of flexibility in respect of costing. Such was the degree of animosity that even getting the interested parties to agree to meet proved a delicate exercise. Within three months cooperation had been secured and most problems were resolved.

Evaluation of all network activities was ongoing, with the member agencies subjecting changes in their performance and in social indicators to the scrutiny of audit committees. For the consumers/clients an annual event was organized with the Better Government for Older People Forums to review progress and to surmount problems.

As a cross-cutting theme, the SPIG recognized this was a pivotally important item for development of an integrated network. There were clear connectivities that needed to be addressed in respect of the correct management of medication, as well as implications for the work of networks; and also in relation to the National Service Framework standards relating to stroke, falls and mental health.

A detailed description of this network's developments, both successes and difficulties, has been written elsewhere [20]. But by way of illustration of the design features set out in the earlier section the following contemporaneous summary can be provided:

> At the network core, a range of practitioners and managers are represented: two community psychiatric nurses (from two NHS Trusts), two district nurses, two community pharmacists (one sits on the Local Health Group Board), two hospital pharmacists, a senior home care manager, a community care manager, a social care team leader, a representative from Age Concern, and a Virtual Organisation Coordinator. The general medical practitioner chairman of the local prescribing group (a statutory body) has connections with the core members.

> In terms of '*approach to integration*', the network core represents the appropriate *range* and *level* of professional and managerial competencies. This network is also especially interesting in terms of 'degree'. Formal organisational integration of all the network roles is not a possibility given this would necessitate a major change in the contractual terms of community pharmacists. In reality, the only possibility of integration is through virtual means as a way of raising the profile of the issue and then as an approach to implementing superior means of communication and co-ordination.

Network governance is maintained through these improved communication and co-ordination activities. The core group members increasingly communicate between themselves outside of the scheduled meetings. For example, a community pharmacist and the Age Concern representative collaborated in a small-scale survey of older people's capacities for following pharmacy advice; this also represents a merging of action research and virtual co-ordination. Using a variety of communications media, including written memos and e-mails, a basis of trust, commitment and mutual respect paved the way for co-ordination. Indeed, using a modified Delphi process, the network core is developing a set of jointly authored protocols that will exercise a system-wide means of control and co-ordination of medication in the community [87].

What the work of this network illustrates is the value of having the neutrality of the white space within which to operate: interorganizational friction could be put to one side during a time of search for creative solutions. But, of course, the solutions themselves could well be capable of causing further friction at the point when action on implementation is required on the part of the participating agencies. The process of 'mainstreaming' the results of the networks' outputs is summarized later and, so, too, the particular role of the SPIG members in achieving this.

The second theme of the work of CHAIN was to explore the role and functions of coordinators in a virtual world.

The Virtual Organization Coordinator (VOC)

This was the third major policy innovation. At the beginning of Project CHAIN only a crude outline existed of the role to be undertaken. The account given below should be seen as resulting from an iterative process of development and review over the life of the action research programme.

The VOC was centrally charged with managing white space activities. What did this entail? That interorganizational and line management are very different became evident. Shorn of diktats, span-of-control and authority, managers of partnerships, alliances and networks require a new toolbox to make things happen. A VOC was created that would serve to deliver CHAIN's aims in accordance with the developing principles of new styles of management. Using and extending, Malone and Crowston's version of coordination, [77] the role was specified as managing (inter-) dependencies in different ways:

Characterizing different kinds of independencies, interdependencies and dependencies.

- Taking stock of organizational and professional interests and connections that determine interactions for a population subgroup; (who is doing what and with whom?)
- Analyzing the stock-take so as to generate a(n) (inter)(in)dependency 'map';
- Giving 'relief' (in the geographical sense) to this map by coding the map with a legend determined by the barriers to integration;

'Characterizing' concludes with a representation of coordination possibilities. That is, with respect to a particular issue, say, medication, there are clear mutual understandings about its underlying nature and logic. Medication issues become framed by the analysis. Outside of the frame lies a set of institutional positions that are not amenable to any immediate change. Inside the frame lies white space territory, open to new coordination possibilities. Of particular importance is the characterization of the different kinds of dependency that are connected with Alter and Hage's [41] quality of relationship. Recalling that network governance operates thorough social mechanisms, the VOC seeks to characterize, for example, 'trust', 'commitment' and 'respect' with a view to harmonizing these as a basis for more technical forms of coordination. Figure 8 summarizes the total range of coordination activity types that aimed to move organizations together and into cooperative, integrated approaches. Several stages are involved.

Identifying Coordination Processes Necessary for Managing

The logic of Malone and Crowston's [77] approach is that different types of dependency (take this to include independency and interdependency) require different coordination processes. Sentiments – trust, commitment, and respect – require different coordination from finance, though ultimately they will need some form of alignment. Faced with the teeming complexity of reality, the trick is to concentrate on key processes that offer a concise way of thinking about actions. In CHAIN, the VOC had a dual approach. First, consistent with an advanced boundary spanning role, the VOC was positioned at the intersection of professional and organizational activity. That is, spanning numerous boundaries creates a *de facto* hub. Second, the VOC was instrumental in creating virtual organizations that would act as, for instance, referent or linking-pin organizations. For example, the VOC was the driving force behind the Strategy and Policy Integration Group (SPIG) which served both to coordinate activities at this managerial level and to legitimize CHAIN activities throughout the partner organizations. This dual approach to agency was both time and context dependent.

In respect of timing, three core processes were considered as critical. When enacted correctly, these processes should generate the necessary white space conditions for further coordination processes. We have postulated these precursor processes as: attracting, guiding, and brokering; and they will tend to occur in this order and represent increasing intensity of activity.

Attracting

By definition, the white space is empty. There is a primary need to get people, activity and resources into the white space. But how do you get something into, and then out of, nothing? The first task of the VOC was to draw or attract people into the white space. Hedberg and colleagues [59] consider attraction as a key management function in virtual organizations. In factoring attraction, they cite both the creating

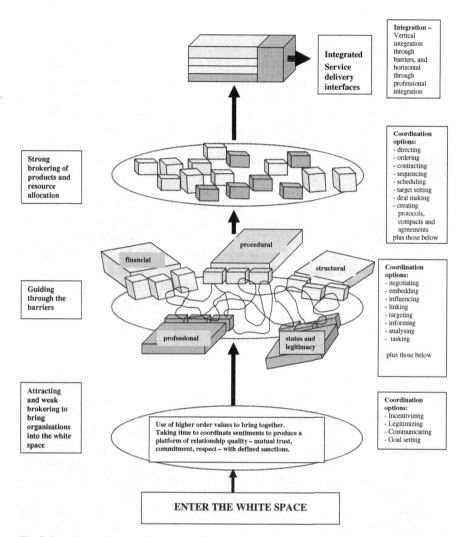

Fig. 8 Developing the co-ordination possibilities of white space – from dependency to integration
Source [20]

of a culture that generates synergies and the transmission of expectations. This latter factor is dovetailed with communicating opportunities, with resonance with our own conception of existing barriers creating an opportunity space. In a sense, marketing is at work here in the form of AIDA – the sequence of Attraction, Interest, Desire and Action that leads from advertising a product to its purchase. The VOC had to incentivize people by giving them good reasons for devoting their time and energy to enter into the white space. Then having secured a level of 'buy-in', the next step is to mobilize and direct action.

Guiding

The choice of 'guiding' to represent the second core process has been influenced by the anthropology literature. What we have termed white space could equally well be described as 'liminal' space. Liminal translates as threshold – a boundary! In anthropology the term was introduced by Van Gennep [88] in association with the three stages of a rite of passage: pre-liminal (cf. preliminary), liminal (during the rite) and post-liminal where the initiate returns to normal reality but transformed. In a series of works, the Turner's [89] developed the notion. Our use stems from the Turners' study of pilgrimage as a liminal state and the role that guides have in assisting pilgrims toward their goal. For our purposes, we required a term that would offer some measure of leadership but without formal command. Clearly, liminal space is largely composed of uncertainty. In CHAIN, we accepted the high level of uncertainty but, equally, it was necessary to convince colleagues that we were not just thrashing around in the darkness. That is, there was direction and purpose, understood by the VOC. There are different types of guiding. We had mountain guiding in mind. A mountain guide will have knowledge of the terrain to be traversed but weather and the composition of the climbing party will be elements of uncertainty. The guide knows the route that needs to be followed but progress, with desired or necessary diversions, will depend on a range of other factors.

Brokering

A fundamental difference between the VOC and typical boundary spanners is the location of the role. To ensure neutrality, the VOC was located within a university department. Fernandez and Gould have identified five types of brokerage relation (see Fig. 9). The neutral location corresponds to the liaison and itinerant broker in the Fernandez-Gould typology. As already stated, these two types correspond to the early stages of white space development when the VOC is communicating with and between partnering organizations so as to 'get everyone on board'. We view this as a weak form of the brokering process. After the guiding phase is complete, in all likelihood, a stronger version of brokerage will be needed in terms of the Fernandez-Gould coordinator. At this stage, brokerage took the form of coordinating the acceptance of agreements or protocols with the SPIG which necessitated thinking about changes in work practices and the re-allocation of funds. Clearly, at this point the barriers to integration may well re-appear, demanding action by SPIG members and considerable brokerage skill on behalf of the VOC. But, with this phase successfully achieved, the move can be made from precursive white space coordination to actual improvements in, say, programme delivery through mainstreaming of the thinking coming from the creative network activity.

Mainstreaming – The Concluding Phase

Earlier, when noting the policy dialog which took place at the preparatory HiAP conference, reference was made to the need many felt for a multisectoral committee/board to be in place at a national level. In the case of CHAIN this was no less

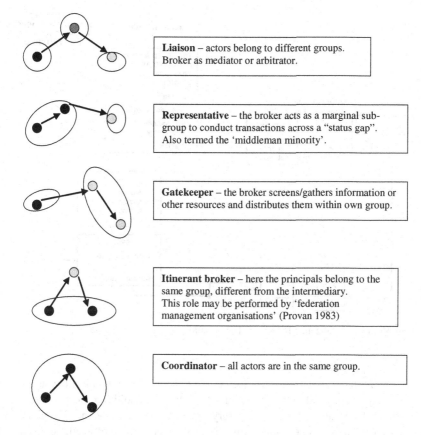

Liaison – actors belong to different groups. Broker as mediator or arbitrator.

Representative – the broker acts as a marginal sub-group to conduct transactions across a "status gap". Also termed the 'middleman minority'.

Gatekeeper – the broker screens/gathers information or other resources and distributes them within own group.

Itinerant broker – here the principals belong to the same group, different from the intermediary. This role may be performed by 'federation management organisations' (Provan 1983)

Coordinator – all actors are in the same group.

Fig. 9 Different types of 'brokerage' Source [90, 91]

true in practice, and was represented by the SPIG, as documented above, working with a Local Partnership Board.

Figure 10, might appear at first glance as a visual representation of the CHAIN design – constructed at the outset and followed as the project model. But this was not the case, although elements of the approach were anticipated, notably the need for a SPIG and the plan for network activity. What was never clear was how the final products of the networks were to become actioned by the participating agencies, that is mainstreamed.

Rather, then, Fig. 10 is the *culminating* statement of how arrangements emerged as best practice which ensured implementation of the multisectoral, interorganizational agenda in respect of the public health of older people. Three key observations can be made:

- Mainstreaming must be thought of as part of a cyclical activity.
- The intent of mainstreaming is recognized at the outset of the cycle, not at the end.
- The process needs coordinating and managing.

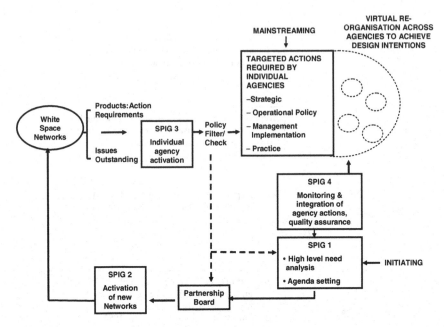

Fig. 10 Virtual reorganization by design: The initiation to mainstreaming process

The SPIG functions varied over the course of the cycle, and their role was critical at each phase, especially given the seniority of the stakeholder representatives. It is the SPIG which carries out the necessary technical appraisal of 'need' and sets an agenda for the agreement of the Partnership Board (a mixture of locally elected and appointed members). SPIG determines what networks are required to occupy the white space and approves their membership to ensure maximum creativity.

As noted earlier the networks are specifically exempted from executive functions and freed from the constraints and limitations that organizational affiliation would bring. Again, then, the SPIG comes into play – receiving the networks' products (and considering outstanding dilemmas), deciding amongst its membership how the required actions will be divided up, and making a contemporary check on the policy milieu to ensure necessary compliance. It focuses on how the 'resources' of each organization, particularly staff effort, will be aligned: this is in contrast to the more anxiety-raising approach of pooled budgets, the mechanisms and difficulties of which have been examined by Durand-Zaleski elsewhere in this book.

SPIG members, as senior officers, do not have to break down any defensive walls as they enter their own organization, but can go in through the doors. They know the organizational DNA, from strategy through to practice, and can 'place' the requirements for action within the existing structures thereby reducing the antibody reactions inherent if internal reorganization was to be proposed. SPIG members, as senior executives of the agencies, have a role in encouraging and sanctioning the formation of the virtual organizations which complete the multisectoral, interorganizational model through virtual reorganization. It is these virtual groups where the real strength lies in achieving change (see Box 3).

Box 3: Virtual organizations

Adaptive and flexible
Cross-functionality and team working
Knowledge understood to be a key resource
Mature approaches to sharing information
Learning organizations
Relational thinking (nonauthoritarian)
Flatter structures

What remains for the governance arrangements managed by the SPIG are the monitoring and quality assurance functions and, above all, performance management of the final stages of the process to ensure needs are being met or, if not, to re-energize the cycle in a different direction.

Conclusion

With this final phase the overall 'policy connect' was complete and the innovation achieved. National level targeting from a number of diverse sectors has been brought together and made operational across multiple sectors at the local level, and on a networked and integrated basis.

References

1. Morgan, G., 1996. *Images of Organisations*. Beverly Hills: Sage.
2. Council of the European Union, 2006. *Council Conclusions on Health in All Policies* (HiAP). Brussels: Council of the European Union.
3. Ståhl, T., Lahtinen, E., & Wismar, M., 2006. *Report of the Policy Dialogues. The Finnish EU Presidency Projects in "Europe for Health and Wealth 2006"*. Unpublished report. Helsinki.
4. World Health European Office, 1984. *HFA by the year 2000: European Regional Targets*. Copenhagen: WHO.
5. Ståhl, T., & Lahtinen, E., 2006. Towards closer intersectoral cooperation: The preparation of the Finnish national health report. In T. Ståhl et al. (eds) *Health in All Policies, Prospects and Potentials*, pp. 169–191. Finland: Ministry of Social Affairs and Health.
6. Sihto, M., Ollila, E., & Koivusalo, M., 2006. Principles and challenges of Health in All Policies. In T. Ståhl et al. (ed.) *Health in All Policies, Prospects and Potentials*, pp. 3–20. Finland: Ministry of Social Affairs and Health.
7. Ritsatakis, A., & Järvisalo, J., 2006. Opportunities and challenges for including health components in the policy-making process. In T. Ståhl et al. (eds) *Health in All Policies, Prospects and Potentials*, pp. 145–168. Finland: Ministry of Social Affairs and Health.

8. Dahlgren, G., & Whitehead, M., 1991. *Policies and Strategies to Promote Social Equity in Health*. Stockholm: Institute of Futures Studies.
9. Swedish National Institute of Public Health, 2003. *The National Public Health Strategy for Sweden in Brief*. Stockholm: Swedish National Institute of Public Health.
10. Agren, G., 2003. *Sweden's New Public Health Policy: National Public Health Objectives for Sweden*. Sandviken, Sweden: Sandvikens tryckeri.
11. Lager, A., Guldbrandsson, K., & Fossum, B., 2007. The chance of Sweden's public health targets making a difference. *Health Policy*, 80, 413–421.
12. Kickbush, I., 2003. The contribution of the World Health Organisation to a new public health and health promotion. *American Journal of Public Health*, 93(3), 383–388.
13. Nilsson Carlsson, I., 2005. In Proceedings of the Interfaculty Working Group on Health Disparities. Cambridge, Mass: Harvard Public Health Now, 18th March.
14. Fine, M., Pancharatnam, K., & Thomson, C., 2005. *Coordinated and Integrated Humans Service Delivery Models*. SPRC Report 1/05, University of New South Wales, Sydney: Social Policy Research Centre.
15. Integrated Care Network, 2004. Change Agent Report 1-12 www.integratedcarenetwork.co.uk
16. Woods, K., 2001. Development of integrated health care models. *International Journals of Integrated Care*. 1. April-June. http://www.ijic.org/archive.html
17. Hardy, B., Mur-Veemanu, I., Steenbergen, M., & Wistow, G., 1999. Inter-agency services in England and the Netherlands. A comparative study of integrated care development and delivery. *Health Policy*, 48, 87–105.
18. Jones, C., Hesterly, W.S., & Borgatti, S.P., 1997. A general theory of network governance: Exchange conditions and social mechanisms. *Academy of Management Review*, 22(4), 911–945.
19. Burt, R., 1992. *Structural Holes: The Social Structure of Competition*. Cambridge, MA: Harvard University Press.
20. Warner, M., 2006. Synergy. In M. Marinker (ed.) *Constructive Conversations About Health, Policy and Values*. Oxford: Radcliffe Publishing.
21. Tillich, P., 1926. Religiöse Verwicklichung. Berlin: Furche Verlag.
22. Tillich, P., 1936. *The Interpretation of History*. Part one trans. By N.A. Rasetski; part two, three and four trans. By Elsa L Talmey. New York and London: Charles Scribner's Sons.
23. Aldrich, H., & Whetten, D.A., 1981. Organization-sets, action sets and networks: Making the most of simplicity. In P.C. Nystrom & W.H. Starbuck (eds) *Handbook of Organizational Design. Volume 1: Adapting Organizations to their Environments*, pp. 385–408. New York: Oxford University Press.
24. Milward, H.B., & Provan, K.G., 1998. Measuring network structure. *Public Administration*, 76(2), 387–407.
25. Powell, W.W., 1990. Neither market nor hierarchy: network forms of organization. In L.L. Cummings & B. Straw (eds) *Research in Organizational Behaviour*, pp. 295–336. Greenwich, Connecticut: JAI Press.
26. Baum, J.A.C., & Oliver, C., 1991. Institutional linkages and organizational mortality. *Administrative Science Quarterly*, 36, 187–218.
27. Grandori, A., & Soda, G., 1995. Inter-firm networks: Antecedents, mechanisms and forms. *Organization Studies*, 16(2), 183–214.
28. Ebers, M., 1997. *The Formation of Inter-Organizational Networks*. Oxford: Oxford University Press.
29. Oliver, C., 1990. Determinants of interorganizational relationships: integration and future directions. *Academy of Management Review*, 15, 241–265.
30. Osborn, R.N., & Hagedoorn, J., 1997. The institutionalization and evolutionary dynamics of interorganizational alliances and networks. *Academy of Management Journal*, 40(2), 261–278.
31. Hannan, M.T., & Freeman, J., 1984. Structural inertia and organizational change. *American Sociological Review*, 49, 149–164.

32. Miles, R.E., & Snow, C.C., 1992. Causes of failure in network organizations. *California Management Review*, 34, 53–72.
33. Ibarra, H., 1992. Structural alignments, individual strategies, and managerial action: Elements toward a network theory of getting things done. In N. Nohria & R. Eccles (eds) *Networks and Organizations: Structure, Form and Action*, pp. 165–188. Cambridge, Massachusetts: Harvard Business School Press.
34. Warner, M., 2000. Health gain investment for the 21st century: Developments in health for all in Wales. In A. Ritsatakis et al. (eds) *Exploring Health Policy Development in Europe*, 86, 236–270. Copenhagen: World Health Organisation.
35. Moreno, J.L., 1934. *Who Shall Survive? Foundations of Sociometry, Group Psychotherapy, and Sociodrama*. Washington DC: Nervous and Mental Disease Publishing Co.
36. Kaluzny, A.D., Zukerman H.S., Ricketts III T.C., & Walton G.B., (eds) 1995. *Partners for the Dance: Forming Strategic Alliances in Health Care*. Ann Arbor, Michigan: Health Administration Press.
37. Curran, C.R., Kuhn, K.W., Miller, N., Skalla, A., & Thurman, R.D., 1999. *Shaping an Integrated Delivery Network: Home Care's Role in Improving Service, Outcomes and Profitability*. Chicago, Ilinois: Health Administration Press.
38. Hage, J., & Alter, C. A., 1997. Typology of interorganizational relationships and networks, in contemporary capitalism In J.R. Hollingsworth & R. Boyer (eds) *The Embeddedness of Institutions*, pp. 94–126. Cambridge: Cambridge University Press.
39. Bazolli, G.J., Shortell, S.M., Chan, C., Dubbs, N.L., & Kralovec, P., 1999. A taxonomy of health networks and systems: Bringing order out of chaos. *Health Services Research*, 33(6), 683–1717.
40. Shortell, S.M., Bazolli, G.J., Dubbs, N.L., & Kralovec, P., 2000. Classifying health networks and systems: Managerial and policy implications. *Health Care Management Review*, 25(4), 9–18.
41. Alter, C., & Hage, J., 1993. *Organizations Working Together.* Newbury Park, California: Sage.
42. Hannan, M.T., & Freeman, J. 1989. *Organizational Ecology*. Cambridge, Massachusetts: Harvard University Press.
43. Rhodes, R.A.W., 1997. *Understanding Governance: Policy Networks, Governance, Reflexivity and Accountability*. Buckingham: Open University Press.
44. Flynn, R., Williams, G., & Pickard, S., 1996. *Markets and Networks: Contracting in Community Health Services*. Buckingham: Open University Press.
45. Mintzberg, H., 1979. *The Structuring of Organizations*. Englewood Cliffs, NJ: Prentice-Hall.
46. Powell, W.W., 1996. Trust-based forms of governance In R.M. Kramer & T.R. Tyler (eds) *Trust in Organizations: Frontiers of Theory and Research*, pp. 51–67. Newbury Park, California: Sage.
47. Gulati, R., & Gargiulo, M., 1999. Where do interorganizational networks come from? *American Journal Sociology*, 104(5), 1439–1493.
48. Bryant, J., 2002. It's all threats and promises: Understanding the pressures of effective collaboration, In D. Purdue & M. Stewart (eds) *Understanding Collaboration, Proceedings of the 8th International Conference on Multi-organisational Partnerships and Co-operative Strategy*, pp. 11–17. Bristol: UWE.
49. Leavitt, H.J., 1965. Applied organisational change in industry: structural, technological and humanistic approaches. In J.G. March (ed.) *Handbook of Organizations*, pp. 1144–1170. Chicago: Rand McNally.
50. Scott, W., 1992. *Organizations: Rational, Natural and Open Systems*. Englewood Cliffs, NJ: Prentice-Hall, Inc.
51. Smith, C., Norton, B., & Ellis, D., 1992. Leavitt's Diamond and the flatter library: A case study in organizational change. *Library Management*, 13(5), 18–22.
52. Homburg, C., Workman, J.P. Jr., & Jensen, O., 2000. Fundamental changes in marketing organization: The movement toward a customer-focused organizational structure. *Journal of the Academy of Marketing Science*, 28(4), 459–478.
53. Duarte, D.L., & Snyder, N.T., 1999. *Mastering Virtual Teams*. San Francisco, CA: Josey-Bass.

54. Ovretveit, J., 1993. *Coordinating Community Care*. Buckingham: Open University Press.
55. Nohria, N., & Eccles, R.G., 1992. Face-to-face: Making network organisations work, In N. Nohria & R.G. Eccles (eds) *Networks and Organizations: Structure, Form and Action*, pp. 288–308. Cambridge, Massachusetts: Harvard Business School Press.
56. Parsons, T., 1960. *Structure and Process in Modern Societies*. Glencoe, IL: Free Press.
57. DSRU, 1998. Towards a common language. Background Paper 2. Devon: Darlington Social Research Unit.
58. Stern, L., 1996. Relationships, networks and the three cs. In D. Iacobucci (ed.) *Networks in Marketing*, pp. 3–7. Thousand Oaks, CA: Sage.
59. Hedberg, B., Dahlgren, G., Hansson, J., & Olve, N.G., 1997. *Virtual Organizations and Beyond*. New York: Wiley.
60. Coase, R.H. 1988. *The Firm, the Market and the Law*, Chicago, Ill: The University of Chicago Press.
61. Lawrence, P.F., & Lorsch, J.W., 1967. Differentiation and integration in complex organisations. *Administrative Science Quarterly*, 12, 1–47.
62. Davis, M., 1983. *Boundary and Space: An Introduction to the Work of D.W. Winnicott*. Harmondsworth: Penguin.
63. Mathiesen, T., 1971. *Across the Boundaries of Organizations*. Berkeley, CA: The Glendessary Press, Inc.
64. Sarason, S., & Lorentz, E., 1998. *Crossing Boundaries: Collaboration, Coordination and the Redefinition of Resources*. San Francisco: Jossey-Bass.
65. Poxton, R., (ed.) 1999. *Working Across the Boundaries: Experiences of Primary Health and Social Care Partnerships in Practice*. London: King's Fund.
66. Aldrich, H., & Reiss, A., Jr. 1971. Police officers as boundary personnel. In H. Hahn (ed.) *Police in Urban Society*, pp.193–208. Beverly Hills, CA: Sage.
67. Aldrich, H., & Herker, D., 1977. Boundary spanning roles and organization structure. *Academy of Management Review*, 77(2), 217–230.
68. Williams, P., 2001. Sieves not shells: Profiling boundary spanners. In: D. Purdue & M. Stewart (eds) *Understanding Collaboration: International Perspectives on Theory, Method and Practice*, pp. 75–82. Bristol: Faculty of the Built Environment, UWE.
69. Williams, P., 2002. The competent boundary spanner. *Public Administration*. 80(1), 103–124.
70. Trist, E., 1985. Intervention strategies for interorganizational domains. In R. Tannenbaum, N Marguiles, F Massarik and associates. *Human Systems Development: New Perspectives on People and Organizations*, pp.167–197. San Francisco, CA: Jossey-Bass.
71. Lorenzoni, G., & Baden-Fuller, C., 1995. Creating a strategic center to manage a web of partners. *California Management Review*, 37(3), 146–163.
72. Human, S., & Provan, K., 2000. Legitimacy building in the evolution of small-firms multilateral networks: A comparative study of success and demise. *Administrative Science Quarterly*, 45(2), 327–365.
73. Emerick, R., Graham, D., & Kovanda, B., 1999. *Multiskilling: Health Unit Coordination for the Health Care Provider*. Albany, NY: Delmar Publishers.
74. March, J., & Simon, H. 1958. *Organizations*. New York: John Wiley.
75. Thompson, J., 1967. *Organizations in Action*. New York: McGraw-Hill.
76. Bolland, J.M., & Wilson, J.V., 1994. Three faces of integrative coordination: A model of interorganizational relations in community-based health and human services. *Health Services Research*, 29 (3), 341–357.
77. Malone, T., & Crowston, K., 1994. The interdisciplinary study of coordination. *ACM Computing Surveys*, 26(1), March, 87–119.
78. Stinchcombe, A.L., & Heimer, C.A., 1985. *Organization Theory and Project Management*. Oxford: Norwegian University Press.

79. Gould, N., (ed.) 2006. *Multi Organisational Partnerships, Alliances and Networks, Engagement*. Proceedings of the 12th MOPAN International Conference, 2005. Devon: Short Run Press.
80. Hamel, G., & Prahalad, C.K., 1994. *Competing for the Future*. Cambridge, Massachusetts: Harvard Business School Press.
81. Bradach, J., & Eccles, R., 1989. Price, authority, and trust: From ideal types to plural forms. *Annual Review of Sociology*, 15, 97–118.
82. Warner, M., 1997. *Re-designing Health Services: Reducing the Zone of Delusion*. London: Nuffield Trust.
83. Warner, M.M., 1999. Virtual reorganisation by design: An approach to progressing the public's health in Wales using networks In *WHO 4th European Consultation on Future Trends*: The Health 21 Framework, London, 14th December.
84. Warner, M.M., 2002. A European view In M. Marinker (ed.) *Health Targets in Europe: Polity, Progress and Promise*, pp.165–180. London: BMJ Books.
85. Warner, M., & Gould, N., 2003. Integrated care networks and quality of life: Linking theory and practice. *International Journal of Integrated Care*. 3 October 9th Edition 2003, ISSN 1586
86. Warner, M., & Gould, N., 2003. Community health alliances through integrated networks (CHAIN): Reporting project progress in South Wales with reference to the UK National Service Framework for Older People. In M. Garcia-Barbela, D. Groen (eds.) *International Conference on New Research and Developments in Integrated Care*. Barcelona: IJIC, 21–22 February.
87. Warner, M., & Gould, N., 2004. Virtual co-ordination: Re-framing systems' management In *Integrated Care Conference*. Birmingham: IJIC, 20–21 February.
88. Van Gennep, A., 1960. *The Rites of Passage*. London: Routledge & Kegan Paul.
89. Turner, V., & Turner, E., 1978. *Image and Pilgrimage in Christian Culture – Anthropological Perspectives*. Oxford: Basil Blackwell.
90. Gould, R., & Fernandez, R., 1989. Structures of mediation: A formal approach to brokerage in transaction networks. *Sociological Methodology*, 19, 89–126.
91. Fernandez, R., & Gould, R., 1994. A dilemma of state power: Brokerage and influence in the national health policy domain. *American Journal of Sociology*, 99(6), May, 1455–1491.

Chapter 6
Knowledge-Centered Health Innovation: The Case for Citizen Health Information Systems

Constantino T. Sakellarides, Ana Rita Pedro, and Manuel Schiappa Mendes

Abstract Twenty first century health systems need to be organized differently – that means around the citizen user. This is a critical change in health governance. It is based on the fact that health is ever more knowledge- and literacy-dependent – and under these circumstances, citizen-centered health information systems, such as electronic personal health information systems, because of their high potential as powerful health literacy tools, are likely to become the sort of innovations that can play a major role in health system change. In fact, the health governance of the future cannot be imagined outside the realm of a "knowledge society," where innovation is a key element.

Innovation refers to ideas, goods, and services, recognized as new and useful, that result from a creative process where knowledge is a key ingredient, implying strong social drivers and producing economic value. In this context it becomes clear that innovation is not, essentially, about technology. It is about creating value in the knowledge society. Some suggest that it is even more than that innovation is "*the* condition of survival in a changing environment.*"*

We are entering an era of massive access to health information, coupled with information-related electronic developments, that brought about the possibility to collected, organize, and use health information intelligently. Consequently, a transition from mass health information consumerism to a mass customization of health information is now taking place. Personal health information records are electronic information resources, owned and managed by individuals with the purpose of assisting them in making health decisions. They are practice-driven innovations, where knowledge is translated into a set of products, services and procedures in a way that is likely to result in health gains, to improve quality of care through better citizen's involvement in the health care process, and to produce economic added value. But personal health information systems are not just about managing health information, they are also a tool for health and digital literacy and citizen's empowerment.

C.T. Sakellarides (✉)
Escola Nacional de Saúde Pública, Lisboa, Portugal
sak@ensp.unl.pt

I. Kickbusch (ed.), *Policy Innovation for Health*,
DOI 10.1007/978-0-387-79876-9_6, © Springer Science+Business Media, LLC 2009

Personal health information systems are innovation systems. They make little sense seen in isolation. Their development is shared by different agents involved as co-producers throughout the innovation process.

The developmental environment of electronic personal health information systems is particularly complex and includes many health systems facets and other relevant societal aspects: technologic markets and platforms, health professional information systems and practices, science systems, local health strategy networks, and health policy and information governance functions.

Currently there are, essentially, four different ways of developing and managing personal health information systems.

Firstly there is the design, production and management of technologic platforms for running personal health records, by industry, serviced directly to the public or through health service partners.

An alternative to industry is a service solution offered to patients by medical associations.

A third possibility is now been provided by health services organization, by including in their health information systems, a virtual space, where citizens might partially access medical health records, and record and manage some of their health information.

A fourth solution, highlighted throughout this Chapter, is that community centred collaborative innovation systems, where a major role is played by personal health information systems users, themselves.

In the context of local health innovation systems, personal health information might become very significant vehicles for more open and democratic societies, where public interest solutions can provide a framework for relating and mutually reinforcing individual and social development on one hand, and the growth of the market knowledge economy on the other.

"Story telling" is an important mechanism for innovation promotion and dissemination.

Selected experiences of real participants (under hidden identities) of a electronic personal health information system project being developed in Barreiro – an old town by the Tagus River facing the city of Lisbon – have been combined as a major, although partial, contributions to the story of Maria Esperança, composed through a future scenario-like exercise. This was developed by this project's management team on the basis of the theoretical references and empirical evidence presented in this chapter.

Health Systems in Transition: Are Health Literacy and Citizen-Centered Information Systems the Critical Change Engines of the Health System?

In the last century it seemed that the protection and promotion of health were straightforward. The premise was that people could be educated to behave in a healthier manner, while public health services would ensure protection from epidemics, environmental hazard, and contaminated water and food. Access to medical care would than take care of most of the rest. On the top of the pyramid there were rational public policies, enjoying political legitimacy, public support, and financing arguments, served by public administrations with clear-cut rules of engagement. This machinery was believed to ensure that policy promises were delivered.

What can go wrong?

It is possibly imprecise to state that the verdict of the last two decades experience was that we were wrong.

Likely, we were just somehow shortsighted.

As Julian Tudor Hart once wrote, "patients are active co-producers of health rather then passive consumers of medical care." Ensuring access to quality health care for all remains a formidable challenge.

Command-and-control organizations, in health systems, failed often on their promises.

Under these circumstances new thinking categories expanded into health systems analysis and terms such as change managing, governance, stewardship, local engagement, information and knowledge management, innovation, health literacy, and citizen's empowerment entered the health policy debate. These new references, now well in their way towards being mainstreamed into the health system's landscape, seem to offer a better way to address uncertainty and complexity in an emerging knowledge society.

Health Systems in Transition and the Citizen

Health systems are slowly but clearly shifting their focus from acute care to long-term care, disease prevention, and health promotion, valuing quality of life.

A large proportion of health care budgets are now spent on a few "chronic diseases" such as diabetes, asthma, congestive heart diseases, depression, and coronary heart diseases. All these require different competences than the ones traditional health care systems used to provide. Beyond biomedical knowledge, organizational, behavioral, information, and communication sciences can contribute to a much more active patient and citizen involvement.

Individualization and a growing number of communities of practice or interest – a new bottom-up health commons – are emerging as major health system's development issues. Genomics, electronic information, and communications systems and citizens/patient-held and citizens/patient-managed health information are contributing to these trends.

Reproductive health continues to be a domain of broad public interest: the public debate concerning abortion takes place in parallel with growing concerns about better and more accessible response to infertility.

There seems to be a new awareness for dealing with the many different facets of violence: Citizen's engagement is necessary for promoting a transition from a disjoint sectorial view of multiple forms of violence to a multisectorial and integrated understanding, in responding to individual, social, and political forms of abuse.

All of these require competent collaborative case finding, action, and follow-up.

Global fattening threats a recession on what has been for many centuries an up-hill life expectancy curve. Public health innovation is focusing on active graying society. Pursuing an intellectually and physically active life, adding life to years, dealing with palliative care, and with assisted death issues poses extraordinary ethical and technical managerial challenges. Only an active public sphere can address effectively such sensitive and complex issues.

Global public health threats, such as pandemics and bioterrorism, seem to require a shift from traditional command-and-control public health emergency approaches to an integrated health governance perspective.

Health services need to evolve are likely to evolve from fragmented, vertical, resource-driven health organizations to horizontal value-based and citizen-driven health networks focused on results. It has been suggested that a fourth "P" – standing for "People" – needs to be added to the often controversial forms of public–private partnerships (PPPs).

From the health financing perspective, there are mounting pressures to evolve from a "traditional welfare" collective approach to one that include investment in human capabilities and looks for a better mix of collective and individual financial responsibilities.

Finally, a clearly observable trend is the transition from provider and management centered health information systems to citizen-centered health information systems.

Citizens' rights and responsibilities toward individual and collective health are beginning to be rewritten.

It has been rightly pointed out [1] that from the 10 recommendations to improve quality of care suggested by the American Institute of Medicine, in 2001 (Institute of Medicine 2001: Crossing the quality Chasm), six are directly dependent on the kind of citizens' involvement that citizen-centered information systems promote. These are continuous healing relationship, customization based on patient needs and values, patient as source of control, shared knowledge and free flow of information, the need of transparency, and anticipation of need.

In this context, citizen-centered information systems, as potentially powerful health literacy tools, are likely to become the type of innovation that can play a major role in health system change – they are likely to be critical change engines in health system's transition.

Figure 1 argues this point in a schematic way.

Health Governance in the Knowledge Society

Aiming to identify the main features of health governance in the 21st century has became a concern of all those interested in understanding and influencing health systems change [2–4].

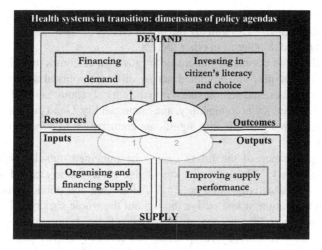

Fig. 1 Health systems in transition: dimensions of policy agendas
(**1**) Traditionally most European health systems are centered on organizing and financing health services supply. This is a powerful agenda with a strong social support and therefore difficult to influence through public policies.
(**2**) Particularly over the last two decades a number of initiatives have been taken to move the agenda from the "resource management" dimension to "service production/outputs" one (Financing/provision split, performance contracting/commissioning, benchmarking). This has been very often a difficult transition since it seems to enjoy a more limited social support than agenda 1.
(**3**) Limited success of the supply side approaches has resulted often in reinforcement of demand side-market agendas (financing demand) through improved enhanced consumer choice, promotion of vouchers and deductibles. In complex health systems consumer-capture by organized interests is a major risk.
(**4**) It is argued that a complex supply–demand mixed agenda will only work for citizens/patients if includes strongly citizen-centered dimensions – improve health literacy and informed choice and representation (agency), though citizen-centered health information systems.

Health governance is about building viable platforms for promoting desirable changes. It is about real, as opposed to formal, decision-making processes on issues of common interest.

Emphasis on the notion of health governance tends to produce two equally desirable effects.

The first of these is a bird's-eye effect, by which the fabric of social interactions elicited by health related interest can be surveyed. The second effect, contrastingly, is an in-depth glance into the community and individual microcosms, where everyday life takes place. Here the real benefits and constrains of what is being decided elsewhere can be felt in more than one tangible way.

Health governance invite us to focus on adding value where it matters the most – the health of citizens and the challenge of realizing each ones well-being potential.

It inquires on what influences health systems evolution, and calls for a better understanding on how health policies work, and on what are the dynamics of key social actors in health systems development;

Moreover, in so doing it touches upon the issue of how health governance relates to overall governance – recognizing the health effects of other policies and also the implication of health policies in other sectors.

Finally the more normative dimension of governance comes into play, as "good governance" principles are promoted across different political agendas and their hierarchies of values, and are translated into the ethical requirements of governance: inclusion, transparency accountability, and contestability. Good governance aims at further democratizing health, as a significant contribution to a more open and less unequal society.

Health governance of the future cannot be imagined outside the realm of a "knowledge society." The idea of a knowledge society is associated with "those knowledge-related activities and policy decisions that add public value ... in the meaningful utilization of knowledge throughout the whole society" [5]. It is therefore important to realize that the notion of knowledge society cannot be reduced to its information technology component. The economy is part of the knowledge society – the knowledge economy influences value-creating processes by fundamentally altering the organization of work, including new forms of cooperation across organizational boarders [6].

The role of knowledge in governance has been enhanced by a more complex and unpredictable world – one of global product chains, where ideas have economic value, and where science and technologic rapid expansion occurs while traditional national, geographic, and political boundaries are under increased challenge [5, 7].

The notion of innovation is a pivotal element of a knowledge society.

Innovation in the Knowledge Society

A few decades ago Theodore Roszak wrote in *Where the Wasteland Ends* (1972) about a young boy and his family waiting for the periodic outburst of Old Faithful the famous geyser in Yellowstone National Park. He describes the excitement and suspense of those gathered around, for the big moment ... silence, then suddenly this visceral murmur coming form mother earth's inner depths ... and than the big white splash high into the air ... and a human uproar of admiration ... an introspective silence ...and amidst the quietness of that special moment, the voice of that young boy, could be distinctively herd: Disneyland is better!

Disneyland! What an unbeatable mix of fantasy and technology!

A New World: Technology and Innovation

Innovation is not, essentially, about technology. It is about creating value in the knowledge society. Some suggest that it is even more than that: innovation is "*the* condition of survival in a changing environment."

The need to look at technologic developments within an innovation framework is a notion of critical importance.

Including technologic progress in an innovation framework is bound to enhance technology's benefits, such as contributing to a better quality of life. It is also likely to avert its unintended negative effects, such as embarking in unnecessary, redundant, excessive, or trivial instrumentation, in detriment of better response to more tangible human needs.

The notion of innovation implies a sense of usefulness and a desire to contribute to a better world. It also means, increasingly, user involvement in creating and delivering new products, services, and processes.

Technology provides tools for better quality of life. Are there circumstances were technologies may be disempowering their users? May we rely on our immediate perceptions or preferred fantasies in dealing with the extraordinary appeal of ever new technologies or is there a need for innovation policies and literacy?

Many our parents or even some of us, first or second generation dwellers of western urban societies, were European very much on the George Steiner's idea of Europe: their were born in a street named after a poet or political leader, they were brought up valuing both Greek classical rationality and Christian brotherhood, their community conscience was exercised in long hours of coffee shop debates or by direct experience of urban and rural landscapes with an human dimension, and have experienced war desperately or its dramatic consequences. They had a sense of tragedy. A sudden end of everything one values could happen.

They came often from large families and tight upbringing, learning, early on, to belong and share, as they left school playgrounds looking for a job.

Most had a profession, even a working place, for life.

They knew their neighbors. All had town squares and identify themselves with a nation state, even when excluded from wealth or recognition. They felt connected to the world through Philips radios and consumed with little guilt and obvious pleasure Nestlé chocolat, collected National Geographic images from paradise, saw World War movies and felt entertained by lighthearted musicals. Choice was limited but borders were clear cut, and right and wrong seemed quite distinct.

They nodded their heads philosophically when confronted with groundbreaking novelties – some from direct experience such as jet planes, televisions sets, insulin, penicillin or the pill, others from distant media echoes of new weapons of mass destruction, rocket journeys towards planet moon or heart transplants. There was a sense of surprise and wonder.

They visited a doctor when they were sick, always prepared for the worst, and shared casually with family and friends the bits and pieces of health and disease understanding these sporadic encounters may have provided. Measles was considered a benign disease, youngsters had appendicitis, sometimes tuberculosis a bit latter, and swollen legs could be either liver cirrhosis or congestive cardiac insufficiency.

As retirement day came along, a grandparent niche was there, warmth on hold.

Than, they would fade away, carried through by intangible forces, coming from far beyond their control or understanding.

Birth may have been problematic – substantial efforts were being made to make it safer – life expectancy was becoming notoriously longer, but death was a destiny to be accepted as it presented itself.

Now it's different.

There is apparently little surprise when one casually finds out that giant containers carriers that can transport 11 thousand containers – each can contain a middle sized car – that turns the transport cost of a pair of jeans from China to England less expensive than carrying it by truck from London to Glasgow. Scaling up transportation volumes from production sites to market places made the difference.

Little wonder.

We have 'rendez vous' in internet chats, engage in virtual shopping, and gift exchanging – "people connecting people." We appreciate Youtube imaging and take risks in Second Life.

We are hypereal.

It seems now possible that sequencing the entire human genome rapidly and at an accessible cost will occur within the next five years. Experts write about "public health genomics" and their relevance to "individual health information management, health policy development and effective health services."

Nestlé focus now on "healthy living" – "good food; good life" has became the Swiss based cooperation preferred image.

Philips is establishing in China, in partnership with Shanghai based Institute of Health Sciences a new health care lab: "early diagnosis and personalized treatment for better health outcomes", is what this is about. Sense and simplicity is their motto.

Web 2.0 is credited for providing a powerful collaborative and interactive space, that enhances a spirit of free and open exchange and sharing among all those that choose to become involved – it is about searching in an almost unending virtual sphere. However where and further delivering a world where one can interact, engage and search, but where Web 3.0, a semantic, highly structured web, is been announced – it seems to be about finding, rather than searching.

These are certainly promising innovations, but apparently unsurprising ones.

They appear to be much more like expected outcomes of scientific and technologic evolution than surprising, astonishing, unexpected, thought provoking, breathtaking, groundbreaking novelties. We seem unimpressed as we adopt constantly new technologies as they hit the market in a continuum of shortening life span for each product generation.

The new is expected. Explanations are not necessarily required.

Some sort of nonchalance towards the new seems unavoidable – unless we become part of it.

Weiser wrote in 1991 about a future world of ubiquitous, unobtrusive, invisible electronic world, that will free man from its tedious common tasks, makings an almost unnoticeable transition from visible, discrete, engaging innovation to immersed, embedded, integrated, and intuitive interfaces.

We are told that "ambient intelligence" experts and investors are carrying through Weiser's vision. Is it reasonable to assume that weak citizen and community participation in the innovation process might often lead to imbedding technologic solutions oblivious of common interest? Does this mean we are than likely to become ever better trained users, while becoming less and less educated in the inner coding that operate our working and living environments?

In the true spirit of modernity, conscious of ones "smallness," is it possible to navigate, engage, self-actualize, and transcend the technologic wonders of this extraordinary new world, thus becoming true partners in the innovation process?

Understanding Health Innovation

The term innovation is frequently loosely used in its common-language meaning as something different than usual – rather than doing more, more intensively, efficiently, or effectively the same.

In a nutshell, innovation refers to ideas, goods, and services, recognized as new and useful, that result from a creative process where knowledge is a key ingredient, implying strong social drivers and producing economic value.

Three different innovation frameworks were selected to address this issue in this context.

Firstly, a public sector innovation framework was extensively developed by the PUBIN (public innovation) studies and publications [8–10], where innovation is seen as set disciplines ranging from economics and management to organizational and systems theories, rather than a formally established theory. It is acknowledged that the notion of innovation comes often strongly associated with its manufacturing legacy – that of a commodity, that is characteristically information poor. Contrastingly, public sector innovation deals predominantly with organizational changes which require a more complex and elaborate understanding/description from an informational point of view.

In this context it is easy to recognize that the fact that innovation takes place within innovation systems is a fundamental idea. Innovation processes encompass different phases, through which "specific behaviors, technologies, and user–producer interactions" are selectively emphasized.

Secondly, a knowledge-centered framework for health innovation has been developed by the Conference Board of Canada, where the innovation process is associated with the creation, diffusion, transformation, and use of knowledge, influenced by environmental cultures, leadership, customer-influenced decision making, standards and regulations, and availability of venture capital and skilled people. Value creation in this process results in improved health systems performance health policies can play here an important role, as they may influence the innovation environment [6].

Finally, National Endowment of Science, Technology and Arts (NESTA) offers a framework for local social innovation, where innovation processes evolve through latent, development, mainstreaming, embedding phases, and changing relationships between authority, organizational capacity, and demonstrable value for the public, as they evolve from one phase to the next one [11].

This model emphasis the fact that local innovation capacity can be improved, by setting up "networks for collaboration, linking people across organizational boundaries to share information and ideas," as well as by the ability of local leaders to address obstacles and opportunities for innovation.

All three frameworks emphasize the fact that the notion innovation systems is of fundamental importance. Innovation systems imply that

(i) Innovation processes take place in specific developmental environments;
(ii) Interaction in innovation's development environments require organizational and managerial arrangements that are centered in innovation drivers and leadership, resource mobilization, and network governance;
(iii) Tangible outputs are created, developed, transformed, mainstreamed, and imbedded throughout the innovation process.
(iv) Innovation added value outcomes can be objectively identified and analyzed.

The additional notions of collaborative or open innovation [12] and of "lead users" of innovations [13], are also of considerable interest for innovation systems, particularly in the case of citizen-centered health information systems.

Collaborative innovation, as opposed to "closed innovation" (innovation is produced internally by an individual company or service and than marked externally), occurs when the innovation processes is shared by different agents involved as coproducers throughout one or more of the different stages of the innovation process.

A particular aspect of collaborative innovation occurs when users themselves contribute to product improvement, including its upgrades and the adoption of possible new usages. These are "lead innovators" or trend setters.

Being innovation a major change engine in contemporary societies, it is relevant to reflect on its public health implications. And it is from a public health perspective that health innovation is here addressed.

In this context it seems useful to look at two key dimensions in health innovation: policy innovation and product, service, process innovation.

They are driven by different kind of social actors. They also differ on the extend they incorporate information and knowledge in the creative process that leads to something recognized as new.

Health Policy Innovations

The health policy dimension (Fig. 2) deals with systems or organizational innovation, and requires translating new ideas in fundamental structural/relational changes, incorporating new performance dimensions with recognizable impact in health systems.

Health policy innovation, driven by a legitimate public authority, requires a major paradigm shift in mind frame, citizen orientation, organizational philosophy in professional contexts, information and knowledge management, outcome orientation, and efficient use of community resources, and is supportive of community-driven innovation.

Over the last quarter of a century, a number of these sorts of innovation can be identified in health systems:

Primary-health-care-based reforms recentered health care systems thinking on peoples needs rather than on expanding use biomedical knowledge and technologies; by emphasizing the importance of service/community interfaces and new professional profiles, they brought about a "health systems renewal"; the health promotion movement was the "next new thing," highlighting now on citizen's empowerment – ideas migrating from political and social sciences were making a recognizable impact on health thinking.

While these developments were taking place a convergent transition on health management and health service organization was occurring – a shift from resource/input and process thinking to a service output and health outcome focus. Value added is seen in "result" terms.

It may be said that the major thrusts of policy innovations, currently, are "citizen centeredness" and the focus in "outcomes/results."

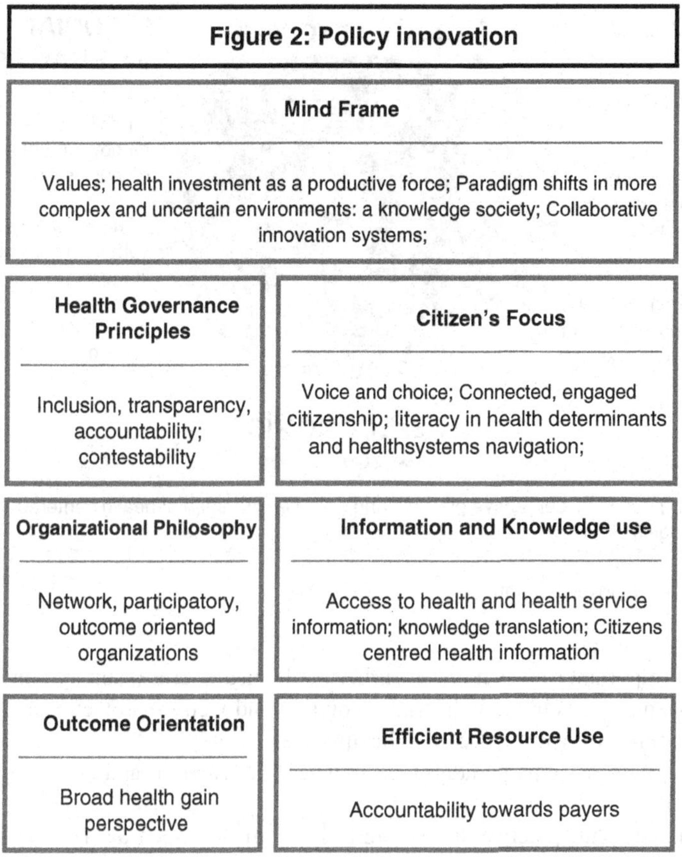

```
┌─────────────────────────────────────────────────────────────┐
│                  Figure 2: Policy innovation                  │
└─────────────────────────────────────────────────────────────┘
```

Mind Frame

Values; health investment as a productive force; Paradigm shifts in more complex and uncertain environments: a knowledge society; Collaborative innovation systems;

Health Governance Principles	**Citizen's Focus**
Inclusion, transparency, accountability; contestability	Voice and choice; Connected, engaged citizenship; literacy in health determinants and healthsystems navigation;

Organizational Philosophy	**Information and Knowledge use**
Network, participatory, outcome oriented organizations	Access to health and health service information; knowledge translation; Citizens centred health information

Outcome Orientation	**Efficient Resource Use**
Broad health gain perspective	Accountability towards payers

Fig. 2 Policy Innovation in health

Ilona Kickbousch sees policy innovation as a way to reorganize how we approach health in the 21st century, essentially through five critical processes: (i) understanding better health as an investment and a productive force in society, (ii) focusing on accountability for health gain, and separate governance mechanisms for health and health care, (iii) increased democratic legitimacy and solidarity in health systems by focusing on ethics and values through a broad dialog with citizens, (iv) move towards broader measures of health outcomes, beyond physical health measures, and (v) engage in network governance.

Practice-Driven Innovation

A second way of looking at health innovation springs directly from the knowledge economy (Fig. 3). It brings health back within a societal context where the economy

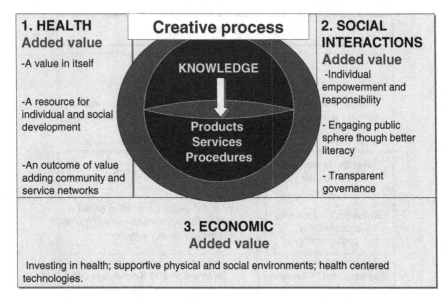

Fig. 3 Practice-driven innovation

plays an important role as it did in earlier public health eras (sanitary conditions of trading-export ports in the industrial revolution and welfare protective and redistribution practices, ensuring access to health care).

It integrates systems paradigm shifts where information and knowledge play a major role.

In this context, practice-driven health innovation is seen as (i) a creative process, requiring imagination and public/private entrepreneurship, (ii) a process that

---

• **Health information platforms for citizens**

Health information resources for citizens through phones or the Internet.
Call centers; Health portals; Internet counseling and other services

• **Health professions support to patient**

Professional health information resources accessible or oriented to citizens.
Patient access to electronic medical records;
Health "information prescribing"

• **Personalized health information platforms**

Tailor made information platforms using ICT devices for providing information at the point of decision

• **Personal health information systems**

A set of health information resources organized and managed by citizens

---

Fig. 4 Typology for citizen-oriented electronic health information systems

translates knowledge into tangible products, services or procedures, (iii) resulting in adding value simultaneously to at least three different domains:

- Health, as value in itself, as a resource for individual and social development, as an outcome of value adding community and service networks;
- Enabling social interactions and individual empowerment and responsibility, by redesigning the public sphere through better literacy, constructive conversations among social actors, and transparent governance;
- Economic growth, trough investing in health, supportive physical and social environments, and health centered technologies.

Again, in all these three domains, adding values means better results – health innovation is "legitimized by results."

Health Innovation Systems

Citizen-centered health information system is likely to emerge as a major health systems change engine. Electronic personal health information systems, owned and operated by citizens, interacting appropriately with their health systems environment (community information resources, professional information systems, and technological platforms) illustrate well the underlying principles of community-driven health innovation – they contribute to better health, change interactive patterns between key health players, have economic value, and are likely to stimulate the appearance of new professions on knowledge translation and brokerage. This is also a privileged area for collaborative (open) innovation and for citizens' involvement, as they assume "lead innovators" roles.

Citizen-Centered Information Systems

Different Contributions Towards More Citizen-Centered Information Systems

People are interested in protecting and enhancing their quality of life, now and in the coming years. Paradoxically, in the "information age," it is increasingly difficult to make sense out of our social and political environment and to relate it with ones' individual, family, and community well-being and aspirations [14, 15]. How to understand a profusely complex environment and harness the personal energy to pilot an hectic daily pace towards realizing our well-being potential is indeed a formidable challenge, even when formulated as somehow incomplete, imprecise, and partially implicit representations. Finding new ways to manage information and acquire knowledge seems, intuitively, an unavoidable path toward better formulating and responding to this challenge.

Over the last decade different contributions aiming at more citizen-centered health information systems can be identified.

A first type, concerned with providing citizens timely health information and orientation – generalist or specialized – is that of health related "call centers." These are now well established, being, possibly, the English NHS direct, one of the better known examples [16]. Interment health counseling and other services are now very prevalent [17].

A second type in this domain is that of health professions support to patients by allowing share, at least partially, their electronic medical records. These records bring together in one single information resource all relevant health information pertaining to an individual patient, that have been originally collected and stored in different health service localities [18, 19].

Another way to support patients is "information prescribing." Here health professionals direct patients (through information prescribing paths) to tailored health information in accessible information resources. The idea is to prescribe information in a fashion very much similar to the way pharmaceutical drugs or lab tests are prescribed, recognizing that information plays a fundamental role in disease cure or prevention, and in health promotion [20].

A third, more uncommon type is that of personalized health platforms that use elaborate ICT to provide citizens relevant information at the point of decision making. An example is PIPS (personalized information platforms for lifestyle and health services support) [21]. This is a particularly elaborate tailor-made information platform designed with the purpose of assisting in making the better informed decisions, form a health perspective, in day-to-day life. It takes into account individual lifestyles, preferences, and health profiles in order to provide, through a variety of ICT devices (mobile phones, PDA, computer screens, and so on), information at the point of decision, weather this is home, the office, restaurants, or supermarkets.

Finally, the fourth type, and closer to the very heart of the notion of citizen-centered information systems, are electronic personal health records or information systems, owned and managed by the individual, interconnected with other relevant information resources in health systems [15].

Personal health record or information systems convey currently an important notion.

They represent a transition from mass consumerization of health information (broad availability and use of health information) to mass customization of health information and knowledge (personalized health information).

Development of Electronic Health Records

The precursors of electronic personal health records (ePHRs) are, of course, familiar personal health files, of diverse shapes and forms, where different kinds of health records are more or less orderly stored.

Then, with the broad expansion of computers (consumer informatics) and growing attention to health literacy and promotion, a large array of electronic health record came to use, progressively substituting "paper" health files.

By electronic personal health record we mean an electronic information resource, owned and managed by individuals, with the purpose of assisting them in making health decisions [22]. In July 2003 Markle Fundation defined ePHRs as an Internet-based set of tools that allows people to access and coordinate their lifelong health information and make appropriate parts of it available to those who need it [23]. In 2005 the American Health Information Management Association (AHIMA) definition of ePHRs adds to the first one key element, some other qualifying features: it is a lifelong resource, universally available, using information coming from health care providers, and the individual. It is also noted that ePHRs need to be maintained in a secure and private environments, its right to access being determined but their individual owner, and recognized as distinct, not a substitute, for legal health care provider records [24].

There are essentially three different kinds of ePHRs, according the variety of platforms. Software programs managed by persons in their personal computers, web-based or in others portable interoperable digital files, to be plugged into a computer, such as smartcard or flash disk. In terms of their content focus ePHRs can generalist – usable by any person independently of health condition and age, or specialized in specific conditions such as diabetes, maternal and child health or heart disease [15, 25].

Some are simple lay-made electronic files; others more elaborated products promoted by health care professionals, health services organizations or commercial vendors. A distinction between electronic health records and health record systems has also been suggested [26]. For reasons of simplicity it was decided not to make this distinction explicit in this text.

In an information age like ours, it might appear somewhat surprising that this trend is so recent and, in most places, for the time being, still far from mainstream health information thinking and practice.

In one's everyday experience there are many opportunities to pick up health information of interest, related to one's own current or past ailments, or those of family and friends. Well-established and respectable disease risk factors such as high blood pressure or cholesterol, the profuse wonderland of human diet, or frequent news coverage of unwilling exposure to chemical, physical, or biological potentially harmful agents attract the attention of many.

Health information comes generously in daily newspaper readings, in generalist magazines or more specialized ones, in an unending number of books and booklets, in TV news, entertainment shows or public service programs, everywhere.

It is well know that for Internet users, health information is at the top of preferred items.

Medical records tend to became increasingly accessible, although at a very slow pace, to patients, and citizens in general.

Health being a matter of such considerable personal interest and there being bits and pieces of health information as a prevailing feature of today's human environment, it is interesting to observe and to try to understand why such a major consumption of health information has generated, up to a very recent past, limited impulses to store and organize at least the more relevant aspects of what is so intensively (voraciously) consumed. Picking up health information so frequently and using to so inefficiently seems a impressively wasteful practice.

However, a closer look at what is involved in achieving a widespread dissemination of this personalized approach to health information reveals a considerable number of important challenges for ePHRs adoption. These have been analyzed by a number of empirical studies [15, 26].

Firstly, there are genuine concerns about information confidentially and the possible misuse of personal information by others, particularly by employers and insurers.

Trust on the safety of electronic records and on those that assist in operating them becomes a critical factor for ePHRs adoption. Elaborate technological solutions to respond to safety concerns have been developing continuously, from different ways of keeping record ID separate from record content to portable electronic keys and different encrypting approaches.

However, these technologic fixes may not suffice, by themselves, to promote the level of trust necessary for expanding citizen-centered health information systems. It is necessary that data protection concerns are not counteracted by policies that adopt higher financial burdens on the basis of personal health attributes – weather disease risk factors, specific lifestyles, or health services utilization patterns.

It is also expected that, as ePHRs move from an initial patchy, quasi-experimental, development phase to later mainstreaming and well-established use, without major, widespread safety incidents, public confidence will be further enhanced [26].

Secondly, there is the question of data accuracy and validation. Unreliable data recording by individuals or inaccurate information from the Internet or any other health information sources imported by ePHRs users seriously affects the integrity for this information resource. It is obvious that less-than-optimal decisions can be taken under these circumstances.

Well-designed and feasible validation procedures are necessary here, on a continuous basis. Also, appropriate glossaries need to be made available to ePHR users to ensure terminological coherence when using or sharing health information [27, 28].

Thirdly, customization, through different building-block combination, allows for choice of alternative pathways in ePHRs development.

Usability studies have stressed the importance of data display and visualization techniques in recalling and understanding the meaning of health information collected and managed through ePHRs. For instance, the degree of complexity and interactivity of ePHRs screens are an important factor in the usability of ePHRs by the aged [22].

Fourthly, organizing and managing health information is possibly one of the most complex undertakings one can experience when comparing it with information management in other domains. The issues involved here a very numerous, often intricately interrelated, and requiring a certain level of familiarity with biomedical and behavioral sciences notions, and some understanding on how health services work. In other words, by calling for some degree of health and digital literacy, ePHRs stimulate and induce progress in these domains [22].

Than, stand-alone ePHRs, operating in an environment where professional electronic health records are not yet widely used and where professional cultures have not fully incorporated the advantages of improved health literacy and patient empowerment, tend to become difficult to manage. Without connecting with reliable sources of information and communicating easily with health care providers, there is limited scope for sustained development for personal health records.

Past economic failure on trying to sell standalone PHR in the US illustrate this point [28]

Another important consideration for ePHRs development relates to the issue of the digital divide and inequality of access to information and knowledge. Elaborate information resources, such as ePHRs, may very well further empower the more educated and economically better-off ones, increasing information and knowledge disparities even more.

There are both good health policy and market arguments for the need to narrow the health and digital literacy divide.

Finally, adopting ePHRs use only makes sense as a lifelong endeavor. This implies a reasonable assurance that ePHRs enjoy a sustainable market from technology operators is of great importance.

Digital preservation, both in content and operational capacities, is a more important challenge that what can be perceived at a first glance [22].

In summary, ePHRs are complex undertaking, highly sensitive to trust, confidentiality and safety issues, requiring validating procedures that ensure the use of accurate data and information. They need to be developed in a customized manner, and be interconnected with other information resources. They are necessarily lifelong endeavors and its use should be accessible to everyone (Fig. 5).

In the US, ePHRs are now rapidly emerging as health information systems components of growing importance. The occurrence, in the aftermath of the 2004

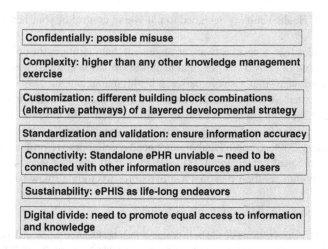

Fig. 5 Electronic health records key challenges: a state-of-the-art summary

Katrina hurricane in New Orleans, of a massive loss of health records in the very circumstance where medical care became particularly necessary was reveling. Katrina Health [29] offered digital PHR to New Orleans residents who wanted it. Since then, the Department of Health and Human Services [30] made ePHRs the cornerstone of the national health information technology strategy (consumer-centric and information-rich health care) [1]. Medicare and Medicaid Services are moving in this same direction. The Department of Veterans Affairs adopted *My Health eVet*. Just a few years ago it was estimated that there were, in the US, more than 60 private ePHR offers [22]. Recent media reports (2008) say that there may exist more than 100 different ePHRs modalities in the US.

It seem that in Europe a major focus on ePHRs development and use is being placed in the citizen's access to medical electronic records [25, 27].

However, currently, in many European countries, different types of ePHRs are being announced, usually through the media.

Enter New, Big Players

The obvious interest, displayed recently, by two technologic giants, Microsoft and Google, in this area, can be seen as significant signs of the development prospects of citizens centered health information systems.

Microsoft has launched "Health Vault" in October 2007. Its presentational text is clear and revealing:

> Welcome to **Health Vault**
> Be well. Protected.
> ... Imagine if you had a way to collect, store, and share the health information critical to your family's well-being.
> **Health Vault** is the new and FREE way to do just that.

Microsoft HealthVault "is designed to put you in control of your health information."

It is includes free-access software arrangement that facilitates the collection, storage and sharing of ones owns personal health information coupled with a choice of services and devices that assist in personal health management.

It is presented as a "hub of a network of Web sites," personal health devices and services including those related to wellness, self-help, disease management, knowledge transfer from science production, and specialized health search engines.

In February 2008, Google Health announced a collaborative project with Cleveland Clinic medical center and 1500 to 10,000 of its patients who volunteered to electronically transfer their personal health records to Google's new health information services.

A related Google statement reads as follows:

> "At Google, we feel patients should be in charge of their health information, and they should be able to grant their health care providers, family members, or whomever they choose, access to this information. Google Health was developed to meet this need"

Although considerably less information is currently available in relation to Google's Health personal health information approach, when compared to Health-Vault, it can be generally described as technologic product (accessible through the Web) that is part of managed information and communication hub linking it to two critical platforms: a "platform of Web services" and "platform of clients" through partnerships with specific health services organizations.

The transition from a personal health record notion to that of personal health information systems as collaborative innovation systems is now becoming more apparent.

From Personal Health Record to Personal Health Information Systems as Collaborative Innovation Systems

Promoting the transition from electronic personal health records to electronic personal health information systems (ePHIS) is of critical importance in perusing citizen-centered health information [26]. Such transition carries far-reaching implications: it broadens the purpose and objectives of earlier ePHRs initiatives, and therefore their usefulness and benefits; it stimulates and explores multiple customized development paths for these information resources; it requires and supports its integration into its community, technologic, health services, and policy environments. This transition also emphasizes the significant difference there is between ready-to-use electronic software aiming at recording personal health information and a community-based customized development projects for personal health information systems.

> *Electronic Personal Health Records (ePHRs)* – This is an electronic information resource, owned and managed by individuals with the purpose of assisting them in making health decisions.
> *Electronic Personal Health Information System (ePHIS)* – This is an "collaborative innovation system" and therefore adds to the ePHRs definition, the notion of a complex, step by step customized undertaking, that requires a continuous interaction with its developmental environment, that plays a major role in promoting health literacy and citizen's empowerment.

Objectives and Expected Benefits of ePHIS

The objectives and possible benefits of ePHIS development are summarized in Fig. 6.

As seen above, ePHRs aim at collecting, storing, and managing, essentially, health care information relevant to the individual. Personal health information

PHIS development objectives	Maslow's classical hierarchy of needs	Info management capabilities
EMPOWERMENT Repositioning in the health system	Self-actualization And transcendence	ADVANCED CITIZENSHIP
HEALTH LITERACY Using information Intelligently in day-to-day health related decisions	Esteem	LEAD INNOVATOR
COMMUNICATION Interacting with others	Belongingness	ORGANIZER MANAGER AND NET WORKER
INFORMATION MANAGEMENT Capturing, annotating, storing and processing data and information	Safety and protection	STAND-ALONE USER
	Basic physiological needs	NON USER

Fig. 6 Individual developmental path in information management and citizen-centered health information systems development objectives in the context of Maslow's hierarchy of needs

systems, while sharing ePHR benefits, perform a broader role: They are communication platforms, not only with health care providers but with any other health information resource that can be of benefit for the health protection and promotion of the individuals concerned; they are likely to become, potentially, privileged, lively, and "self-transforming" tools for health literacy – improving ones capacity to use information intelligently in day-to-day health-related decisions. By organizing and managing relevant health information, providing an effective communication and networking platform, and promoting health and digital literacy, ePHIS display considerable potential to reposition people in their health systems by empowering them with "voice and choice" in individual and community health maters.

The health literacy and empowering potential of ePHIS in assisting individuals to realize and achieve their well-being capacities may be argued both theoretically and empirically. In fact, this sort of progression parallels well with what might be the expected progression on one's hierarchies of need – as recognized by Maslow as far back as 1943. It also goes well along the lines of personal development concepts, toward lead innovators and advanced forms of citizenship.

Personal Health Information Systems as Customized Developmental Undertakings

The notion of PHISs as complex customized developmental undertakings is of fundamental importance. It is based on the requirement and expectation that each one defines the content and ordering of the building blocks necessary for progressing in health information management and in health and digital literacy.

Customization of ePHIS development means, basically, path-finding through incremental steps what sort of building-blocks combination better corresponds to ones personal characteristics and preferences.

In order for this to happen, a number of factors need to be taken into account.

It is naturally important to start with the simpler ePHIS building blocks or those perceived by the individual as been more necessary ones (recording pharmaceutical drug taking history and adverse reactions, or information useful in case of emergency), and progress towards more complex ones, at a pace fitting individual objectives, abilities, availability, and commitment. It is also useful to consider that there are occasions when persons are particularly open to adhere to health information management practices, as it is the case at the inception of chronic illnesses or when the need to support illnesses of close relatives is more acutely felt.

In anticipating ePHIS management by citizens, it is necessary to take into account what people do in their day-to-day activities. In fact, it has been pointed out that while professional work flows tend to be studied, this in not yet the case in relation to persons in their usual environment, where their flows are poorly understood [28]. As indicated above, usability aspects are important. Here, particularly age-related aspects of usability require special consideration. Building-blocks configuration can take many different shapes and forms. Figure 7 illustrates one of all such possibilities.

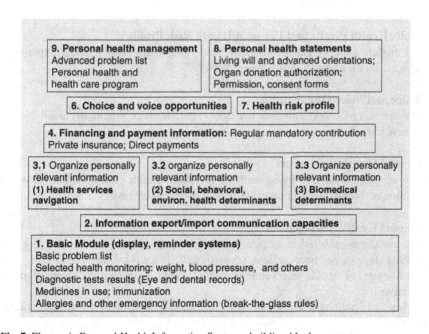

Fig. 7 Electronic Personal Health Information Systems: building-blocks contents

The underlying logic of this particular design can be summarized as follows.

Basic Module
This basic module is for everyone's use, either as a definitive solution or as a starting point for further development. It includes information for medical emergencies. Different display and reminder systems can be incorporated. It may contain a basic health library. Its contents can be totally or partially shared through printouts.

Information Export/Import Communication Platform
This is a communication module, which functional capacities may go from a simple e-mail communication mode to much more elaborated ones (personal Web page function, networking and community of practice functions, link to the i-citizen Web page).

Three modules are available for recording personally organized information on *health services* (related to ones own community health services), *biomedical* (including genetic) *determinants, and social, behavioral, and environmental health determinants.*

Financing and Expenditure Information
This module records financial commitments in relation to health promotion and health care (stimulating the analysis of alternative options) and takes stock of all health related expenditures.

Family Health Profile and Personal Health Risk Profile
This module summarizes information concerning one's family health experience and what might be one's health risk profile.

Choice and Voice Opportunities
Here are recorded opportunities (already experienced or potentially available) to improve choice or express views on ones health system.

Personal Health Statements
Such statements include living wills or advanced health care orientations, organ donation authorization, and permission or consent statements.

Personal Health Management
This module is centered in a "personal health plan." The rational underlying this health plan can be more or less sophisticated. It may include notions of cost-effectiveness of health interventions and of health impact assessment of other initiatives.

Here, it is important that the design, content, and ordering of the different building blocks are clearly presented and understood by the potential users so they choose, in an informed way, a preferred development path.

Personal Health Information Systems as Collaborative Innovation Systems

Citizen-centered health information systems are innovations systems of great public health interest.

They make little sense seen in isolation.

Personal health information systems are tangible, renewable products of an innovation process taking place in a specific developmental environment.

They are local collaborative innovation systems as their development is shared by different agents involved as coproducers throughout the innovation process.

They stimulate lead innovators as some end users tend to become very actively involved in the innovation process.

The developmental environment of ePHISs is particularly complex and includes many health systems facets and other relevant societal aspects [31].

Some of these are highlighted here (Fig. 8): technologic markets and platforms, health professional information systems and practices, and science systems, local health strategy networks, and health policy and information governance functions.

Technologic Platforms

Although it is important to re-emphasize that citizen-centered information systems are essentially not about technology, all ePHIS are dependent on the technologic

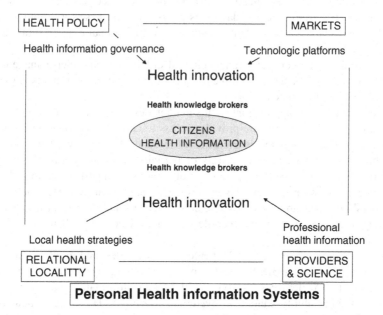

Fig. 8 Context integration: personal health information systems as collaborative innovation systems

platforms that operate them. These tend to evolve at an extraordinarily rapid pace. As referred to above, ePHIS are lifelong endeavors: once one organizes health information electronically, it is reasonable to expect that the technologic devices that operate them evolve in a sustainable way, so one can be confident that operational and financial discontinuity in the access and use of the appropriate technology will not occur.

This requires from ePHIS supporters and promoters a prospective attitude toward technologic markets in this domain. It is important to know what is currently being offered, how these offers will evolve in the near and more distant future, and, as far as one can know, what is happening in the technologic pipeline.

Professional Health Information and Science Systems

Electronic health records, eHRs, for professional use are known since the 1960s.

There is little doubt that these will become mandatory technical and ethical requirements of good medical practice and quality health care in the very near future. It is, however, necessary to gain some insight on their adoption challenges. Key issues for success in professional working environment seem to include such diverse factors as sources of financing, operational requirements (interoperability, standardization and connectivity with other information systems), redesign of workflow in the organization, and support in enhanced team work and management of change.

The usefulness of these electronic health (medical) records goes beyond clinical practice. Electronic records databases provide a solid base for "rapid learning health systems" that can complement randomized trials in building up future health knowledge bases [32].

The need to interconnect citizen-centered ePHIS and provider-managed eHR seems obvious. In fact, a considerable number of initiatives have been taken to build ePHR by accessing existent eHR.

There are concrete applications, in the market, designed to provide both the common citizen and the health care provider access to common information resources, each one of them accessing it from their one coded entry points, but having the possibility of allowing access, entirely or partially, to their records, under specified conditions. Of course, transparency is of paramount importance here – recorder holders are kept informed on who accesses what and when [24]. Here health care providers' concerns about the possible consequences, and their legal implications, of using inaccurate information recorded in ePHIS need to be taken seriously into account.

Also, it can be observed that the perceptions, attitudes, and mind-sets of health professionals toward ePHIS vary extensively in the field. The traditional asymmetry of patient–provider roles vis-à-vis health literacy, information management, and decision-making ability cannot be overcome overnight. These are critical issues that need to be managed sensibly. The current shift from acute to chronic-diseases-centered health systems may be helpful in this regard.

It may be argued that a sensible development course of action in this domain could be to focus the necessary technical and financial resources in mainstreaming electronic medical records and then, as second step, gradually granting access to patients and citizens to these records. This could than be the starting point of the personal health information system's expansion.

However, there is currently a clear ongoing cultural shift toward intensive use of health-related information by citizens, and the fact that citizens and professionals manifest different underling logic in organizing their health information is now better recognized [28].

Science systems play here also an important role. Knowledge is the basic business of personal health information systems – their operational currency. Therefore, ePHIS depend on knowledge translation as "the synthesis, exchange and application of knowledge by relevant stakeholders" in order to ensure the reliably of their information contents.

In a recent WHO report it is stated that "bridging the know–do gap is one of the most important challenges for public health in this century . . .knowledge translation strategies can harness the power of scientific evidence and leadership to inform and transform policy and practice . . . policy-makers, health workers, researchers and the community can work together and share experiences and lessons in bridging the gap" [33].

Personal health information systems are becoming a critical part of health systems knowledge value chains aimed at delivering added value for citizens by improving access, quality, and efficiency of health care services and producing better health outcomes.

They are already becoming become an important part of the knowledge economy.

Relational Localities and Local Health Innovation Systems

As observed above, citizen-centered information systems need to be customized, meaning that they need to fit the personal characteristics of its holder. It may now be added that they also need to fit the holder's local, physical, social, and cultural environment.

This poses many challenging questions.

Can one make the case of local versus global evidence in built-up personal health literacy resources and supporting local deliberative processes?

There seems to be a reasonably broad agreement that evidence is context sensitive and that of good "global" evidence must be triangulated with reliable local knowledge.

Information on prevailing health risks (from air pollution to hazardous locations and accident-prone areas) need to be locally produced and disseminated to personal health information systems. It is expected that the adoption of ePHIS in any locality, at a considerable scale, will place added pressure on the availability and accuracy of locally generated health information. Consequently, local health strategies can find here a new and very meaningful challenge, and would be probably well advised to look at the development of citizen-centered health information systems as one of their most significant operational targets.

Relational localities inherent in ePHIS development certainly require intelligent and demanding engaging strategies and persistent social entrepreneurship. Key elements in collaborative innovation systems, such as electronic personal health information systems, are engagement at the local level [34, 35], knowledge translation, and knowledge brokerage.

Warner and Gould [36] indicate that intersectorial engagement at the local level requires elaborated network governance to operate effectively in the neutral interorganizational "white space" territory. They suggest that for operating in this territory, a set of functional arrangements – "virtual reorganization by design" – are necessary. A critical role in ensuring this sort of virtual reorganization is to be played by coordinators competent to " . . . colonize the neutral territory, to cross organizational boundaries, and to broker action within the mainstream operations of participating bodies."

A wide range of channels of engagement – technologies of connection – are currently available. These provide almost endless possibilities of public communication which is interactive, inclusive, relatively cheap to enter, and unconstrained by time and distance [35].

Health Information Governance

Well-informed decisions are desirable at all health systems levels, everywhere: by policy makers, public health practitioners, managers of health service organizations, and health care professionals. This naturally is also true for community leaders and citizens.

Health information governance is becoming a major component of health policies.

It is necessary to ensure that accurate, timely, relevant information is accessible to all that need it, when they need it. Relevant health information should flow to known decision-making hubs, transparently and safely, through interoperable IC technologies. This is expected to take place in a way that respects information confidentiality, builds trust, and produces added value to health and to the quality of social interactions.

Good health information governance is currently a major theme for public health innovation.

In this context, it is important to map citizen-centered information systems into the developmental strategies of health information infrastructures and functional requirements.

Can we find them there? To what extent do health policies and health information governance recognize and value the potential role of ePHIS in health promotion and improved quality of care? What are, for each specific cultural milieu, the obstacles and opportunities for promoting citizen-centered health information systems?

There is no "citizen centeredness" without finding out about citizens' views.

Surveying, and taking into account, citizens' views and expectations concerning health information must become a key element in good health information governance.

Over the last few years, considerable information, from a variety of different sources, has became available on how people feel vis-à-vis organizing, storing, and using personal health information.

Two Markle Foundation studies in 2005 found that 60% of those surveyed support the creation of a secure, personal health record and showed that the majority would be comfortable with ePHR use particularly for pharmaceutical drugs prescriptions (fill and check), for accessing test results from the Internet, for checking mistakes in medical records, and for e-mail communication with their doctors [37].

Harris Interactive online polls have been taking place since 2004, covering various aspects of health information use. In a more recent poll, implemented by this same organization, for the Wall Street Online Health Industry Edition, in late 2007, surveying 2,153 US adults, it was observed that 26% of those surveyed said that they were using some kind of eHR, mainly the one kept by their physician. Only 33% of those surveyed were very confident that health care providers had a "complete and accurate picture of their medical history" – that percentage increase to 50% for those having access to medical health records.

The Eight European Counties Survey on the Future of Health, which includes Germany, Italy, Poland, Slovenia, Spain, Sweden, Switzerland, and United Kingdom, also illustrates the importance European citizens attribute to their role in health information management [38]. When those surveyed were asked to value different sorts of innovation – consultation by phone, telemedicine, having access to their health information in an electronic way, having available information about providers to choose based on this data, or having consultations more quickly but without assurance to see the same doctor – they valued the most the possibility of managing electronically their health information (Smartcard).

Alternative Configurations for Electronic Personal Health Information Systems

Currently, at least four different approaches for developing and managing electronic personal health information systems may be identified.

Firstly there is the design, production and management of technologic platforms for running personal health records, by industry, serviced directly to the public or through health service partners. This has been mostly the experience of electronic health records developmental, and it is also the case for the personal health information systems, now been launched by major ICT developers, as indicated above

An alternative to the service solution offered by ICT industries, is exemplified by the Canadian Medical Association that offers a electronic health information system that allows patients to organize and manage their own health information, and facilitates its communication with their physician.

A third possibility is now been provided by health services organization (England, Germany, Austria, Portugal) by including in their health information systems, a virtual space, where citizens might partially access medical health records, and record and manage some of their health information.

Finally, a fourth kind of solution is related to what has been above designated as "community centered collaborative innovation systems". Although this conceptual construct is in an early developmental stage, it may carry far reaching implications for health literacy, community development and innovation, and citizen centred health systems [39,40].

It is here suggested that local collaborative innovation systems (LCIS) for personal health information development can be characterized as follows:

(i)   Networks of personal health information users, originating from some sort of consumer/patient association, constitute the core element of LCIS.

(ii) Health information users are involved in the design and implementation of openly accessed technologic platforms that allows for a step-by-step, customized development of personal health information systems, including the selection of added public and/or market knowledge servicing.

(iii) Health information related LCIS pursue actively ways to ensure effective communication and cooperation with local health professionals and services, both in personal care and in public health.

(iv) Citizens-based consultative and support structures are organized, aiming at improving health and digital literacy, knowledge translation initiatives from science systems, and at providing assistance in making intelligent market choices on health information offers.

(v)   New kinds of expertise are stimulated through LCIS, such as those of "health information brokers", capable of contributing to information content quality, trust on confidentiality, and easiness with information and communication technologies.

(vi) Funding strategies are likely to encompass two different modes - a "start-out mode" (which may include a mix of public development funds, social non-for-profit organizations, "social responsibility" funds) and a "sustainable" mode dependent on the value patterns created during the start-out mode.

The LICS approach may play an important role in averting the establishing of deeply rooted embedded dependences in personal health information systems. These can happen when personal health information systems are thought out just as simple extensions of electronic medical records, or when they became part of tightly integrated ICT platforms, difficult to track, disentangle and influence

In the context of local health innovation systems, personal health information might also become very significant vehicles for more open and democratic societies, where public interest solutions can provide a framework for relating and mutually

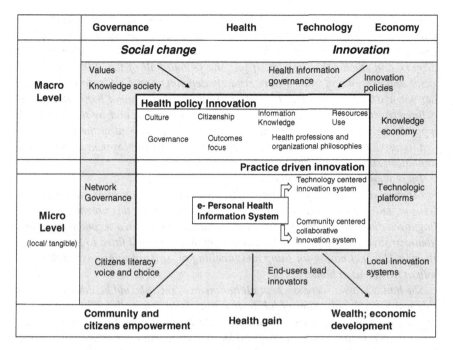

Fig. 9 Conceptual mapping for innovation on citizen-centered health information system

reinforcing individual and social development on the one hand and the growth of the market knowledge economy on the other.

Personal health information systems face a challenging developmental path: one with personally and sensitive issues, interacting with a formidable mix of systems complexity, a playing field of many diverse interests, a very broad scope of health scientific knowledge, professional perceptions and codes of conduct, and a large variety of more or less subtle technology embeddings.

Figure 9 displays a summary conceptual mapping for innovation on citizen-centered health information systems. It is based on the different innovation frameworks surveyed in this chapter, as well as on the experience gathered through the action research project briefly described bellow. It highlights the convergence of theoretical notions from different origins, into the developmental environment of personal health information systems.

The Story of Maria Esperança

In the mid 60's, Maria Esperança, aged 9, settled, with her older brother, in a small town called Barreiro, across the Tejo (Tagus) river from Lisboa, where he found a job in a large industrial chemical complex called CUF.

In mid XIX century the town of Barreiro was adopted as the railway terminal of the growing railways network south of Tagus river. Its proximity to the country capital in addition made, made it attractive to industrial settlements, in particular cork and chemical industries. If fact the second half of the 1900's Barreiro's social and economic fortunes were strongly dependent on CUF's development. In fact when CUF came to this town in 1907 there were around 8.000 inhabitants in Barreiro. Only 30 years later this number had tripled, and by the early 80's, approximately 90.000 people lived there. However, by the end of the next decade, post industrial times were reshaping life in Barreiro. Unemployment increased and population started to decline steadily.

There were difficult times ahead.

Esperança married early, with a CUF worker, and soon after, they had their first son, Diogo. A few years later Maria was born. During this pregnancy she was diagnosed diabetes. Meanwhile Esperança started working in a secondary school as administrative staff, at the library. This occupation was well fitted to her organized lifestyle. Her inclination for filing and labelling all sorts of things was well known both at work and at home.

She had a drawer were she kept all her medical records and health information. This was quite a collection of lab tests result sheets, typically unfitting Xrays (in size and shapes) from earlier years, yellowed personal notes, doctor's appointment records, used pharmaceutical drugs folded packages and their information inserts, immunization and blood type record, past pregnancies and old child's growth curves and baby clinic booklets, health service bills, photocopies of newspaper and magazine articles, concerning diet, sexuality, sleeping disorders, physical fitness programs, environmental and food hazards, and the latest on the flu pandemic alert popular literature.

She used to call it my "health archives." Everybody else in the family knew it as another of Mom's paper drawers. Nevertheless, it was a fact that, in numerous occasions, Esparança's rudimentary archives proved very useful in responding to their GP need to recall past health experiences in dealing with current illness episodes.

Life went on in Barreiro.

Esperança's family, with small salaries and occasional unemployment episodes, maintaining basic household commodities and educating their children, barely could make it economically. As was also the case for many other women in her social condition, life was tough. As a working spouse and mother, going through heavy daily routines, she had little or no time for herself.

Days were long, and nights even more monotonously alike, one after the other.

Many years went by with almost no opportunity to think on her own development needs as an individual.

Often Esperança recalled, somehow sadly, her school days, the encouragement she often got from the best of her teachers, as their recognized on her an inquisitive and creative mind.

So many unfulfilled promises!

One day, while talking with a friend, also a diabetic, Esperança found out about a new project being initiated at the Diabetics Association aiming at helping people to organize their health information. When visiting the Association, a few days later, after working hours, she was surprised to find some of her neighbours sitting in newly installed computer room. They had the assistance of a young woman, hired to help improving digital literacy for those interested in participating in this citizens centred health information project known as "i-citizen"

It became immediately crystal clear to her what these people were up to! They were using computers to live up all paper filled "health archives" like hers!

She signed up. Their children have grown up. She had more time now.

Barreiro's i- citizen project

This Diabetics Association in Barreiro has approximately 1050 members. Approximately 600 are actives ones, and about 65% have diabetes. The main objective of this Association, beyond supporting diabetics, is health promotion. It provides its members to low cost services on psychology, nutrition, and podiatry services.

In partnership with this Diabetics Association, Barreiro Primary Health Care Center, Regional Health Administration and General Direction of Health, the Portuguese School of Public Health is developing, since early 2007, a project aiming at developing and evaluating a citizens centred health information system (i-citizen project), which main objectives are: health information management by citizens (storing and processing data and health information), enhancing electronic communication capacity (the interaction with the others, namely health professional), promoting health literacy and citizen's empowerment.

Project development steps

1. Health and digital literacy survey for members of Barreiro's Diabetes Association: This is basically a base line assessment of literacy levels (220 surveys by postal questionnaires, with a response rate of approximately 50%).

2. Program for improving digital literacy: in order to assist those with low digital literacy levels, a small "digital lab" was installed in the Diabetics Association. An "information assistant" is available to help improving digital literacy for those interested in participating in this project. He keeps a "health and digital literacy diary" were highlights of this experience are recorded.

3. An electronic personal health information prototyped: This was designed to perform as a learning toll for citizens, as they experience

different health information managing "building blocks", while progress
in health and digital literacy.

4. Personal health information system's performance as an innovation sys-
    tem: This phase is taking place in the first semester of 2008, and implies,
    essentially, surveying and assessing the development environment of
    personal health information systems - attitudes and perceptions of health
    professionals, future prospects of technologic platforms being developed
    in this domain, links with local health strategies, and contextualization
    in national, regional and local health information governance

This is an action research project aiming at promoting and studying electronic personal health information systems as "community centred collaborative innovation projects".

*During the projects workshops many examples were given as to the usefulness of
these computerized systems:*

*There was the story of a 79-year-old lady with diabetes and congestive heart
failure that was one evening rushed to an emergency department. Asked about her
medication, she could not really remember any detailed but was able to give to the
attending physician her electronic personal health system password. There he found
that she was allergic to the aspirin he had just prescribed. He was able to correct
it, and avoided a major problem.*

*Another example of an effective ePHIS user is that of a person that has her test
results electronically transferred to her own information resource, and uses a website to find out what the results mean. She is also able to contact electronically her
primary health care physician for advice or appointments. Furthermore she has
permission to enter her aged mother ePHIS and helps her in complying with her
medication schedule.*

*There was also the account of a man in a comatose state is delivered to an emer-
gency room, without information on the possible causes for his condition. However
the attending physician was able to access his medical history through an ePHIS
found out that he had diabetes and was therefore able to initiate immediately a
life-saving treatment.*

*These advantages were almost intuitive for her. At this stage, however, she had
some concerns about the systems' ability to secure confidentially. She could not
judge fully for herself the technicalities of such concepts as "keeping citizens identity separate form data" or "encrypting." She felt it was important to keep trying to
sort these things out. It wasn't very comfortable to her to settle this issue on faith.*

*Esperança was asked to fill up a questionnaire aiming at assessing her health and
digital literacy. She was encouraged by the fact she had done so impressively well
in this kind of test about her health knowledge and was not discouraged by her low
marks on digital literacy. To the contrary – this was a stimulus to take full advantage
of the learning opportunities being now provided at the Diabetics Association.*

It was relatively easy for her to get a good hold onto the basic module of "i-citizen." After all it was essentially a matter of inputting into this software information she had been storing and organizing for many years. The next step for her was to become familiar with the communication module.

Buying a home computer became o new household budget priority. They found out that this could be subsidized through a government programme aiming at promoting digital literacy in the country

One afternoon she decided to surprise her GP, by displaying an i- citizen print out showing her usual test results, her weight and blood pressure curves, as well as her current medication schedule. Although he was familiar with the i-citizen project, he didn't expected it could progress so rapidly. They agreed to start communicating from Esparança's i-citizen to the GP's electronic health record and vice-versa.

From here Esperança progressed rapidly to the other building blocks of i-citizen. As this progress was taking place, something new stared happening.

i-citizen program managers select a group of users for a more in-depth interview as part of i-citizen first performance evaluation. For Esperança, one of the selected users, this was a surprise – outside her inner circle of family and friend nobody as ever expressed much interest in her views.

This was however a very welcomed exercise since she has indeed some ideas on how to make this tool even more user friendly and how to improve the i-citizen library component in order to make it more easy to consult. Her experience at the school library finally proved useful some where.

i-citizen program managers were very impressed by the quality of the views and suggestions they could get from some of the users, Esperança included. They decided to select six of them as permanent project part-time user-consultants.

Esperança was enthusiastic.

She invited the others to an after dinner "rendez vous" to discuss their new role. They found these exchanges fruitful. These became regular meetings. They begin searching in the Internet for thoughts on the kind innovation they were experiencing. They got some help for improving their English proficiency. One evening one of them arrived particularly excited, waving a few pieces of paper in her hand. "This is it" she proclaimed, and handed out a few selected pages of Eric Von Hippel "Democratizing Innovation." There were moments of silence, as the group read a couple of paragraphs, marked in yellow. Suddenly one of them of them exclaimed: "we even have a name – we are lead innovators." This turned to be a long exciting evening.

Esperança deployed her modest celebration "kit": a few slices of bread from their neighbourhood's baker and of cheese from an Azeitão, a generous serve of olives from Elvas, a small taste of an excellent red wine from Alentejo.

Back home, spouses were surprised by everybody's late, late arrival.

Next meeting there was even more to talk about. New terms, new concepts had been emerging through their readings – collaborative innovation, open innovation were notions they were eager to grasp appropriately, by discussing their readings and how they applied to their experience in i-citizen. But the best piece of news that evening was the fact that some of them have been successful in their application to become information assistants in the Internet access points, made available in many of the municipalities of that area. Now they had an expertise that was becoming socially recognized. This did a lot for their self esteem.

But there were also difficult circumstances, as well as some creative moments. In one occasion, during a meeting with some beginners in ePHIS use, there were tense moments. One of them appeared clearly uncomfortable with the prospect of sharing some of his personal information with more experienced colleagues, even as part of a learning exercise. Although this was a misunderstand – no such sharing in fact was happening outside a specific request for assistance in a particular aspect of the personal information system by an interested party – it raised a key issue in any collaborative experience: trust.

That afternoon Maria Esperança could observe how trust was something one can clearly fell or not, but how difficult it was to reasonably converse about it. But ingenuity can be wonderful – next meeting a member of the group came wearing a t-shirt were it could be red: "You can't hate someone whose story you know." She got the idea late night, by e-mail, from a friend that happened to be reading Margaret Wheatley's "We Are All Innovators."

Many of them felt that this form of indirect communication could work and clear the air gracefully, in delicate circumstances. They decided to use it more frequently.

One more year went by.

i-citizen was now expanding rapidly to other patient associations, municipalities, and even a nearby "health cities project." Esperança's group was called to help in the development of these projects. As this work became too demanding for a such a small group, they start contacting interested users from these new i-citizen spin offs in order to expend their working capacity. Few months later they ended up with an i-citizen collaborative network, which included a community of practice component that assisted in sharing their experience based learning. They now realized, thrilled and somehow worried, that have begin in fact to manage a virtual organization supporting citizens to develop their health information systems and interacting with program managers, public health authorities, health service managers, and software producers to covey user views on electronic personal health information systems development.

Than a big step forwards was about to happen.

The Regional Health Administration of Lisbon opened selection procedures for "health information brokers" to assist the development of i-citizen in the Region. To those selected an on service training on health information brokering will be offered by the National School of Public Health in Lisbon. Many of the network member, those looking for a new profession on citizen's centred health information, applied. Esperança is among them. They are very confident they are going to be selected.

What whatever the selection results might be, they are now more knowledgeable and confident citizen, trusting that other opportunities will emerge.

In fact, in the lat few months, there have been some signs that might point to a Barreiro renascence: The new airport serving the Lisbon metropolitan area is going to be developed not far from Barreiro; a third bridge linking the northern to the southern of the Tagus River may very well be a Lisbon-Barreiro bridge. New communication infrastructures linking this town with other urban centres in the southern bank are been planed; old decayed industrial facilities, abandoned a few years ago, are been looked with renewed interest by investors. As the railway terminal, 150 years ago, these new infrastructures were expected to bring to Barreiro a new era of prosperity.

In Maria Esperança's circle there is both excitement and apprehension about these new developments. Would the new jobs (or the best part of them) to be created benefit predominantly the local community or would they be in fact taken over by newcomers? It is apparent to them that a possible new Barreiro boom, unlike the one experienced during the first half of last century, will be very much centred in 21st century service organizations.

Was Barreiro prepared for local innovation at a larger scale, implying new rules and tools for social engagement, new ideas and elaborate, demanding network governance?

One evening three was a large gathering at City Hall to discuss the future.

Maria Esperança couldn't resist and gave some inspiring international examples she had selected from the last NESTA report, just published, and entitled significantly "Transformers" [11].

She was interrupted abruptly by a sharply dressed gentleman, sitting not far from the Mayor: "you people" he said angrily, "keep coming up with these odd imported stories from foreign places that have nothing to do with our Barreiro," and added, even more loudly – "we will fail to take any advantage from these new opportunities if we loose our senses altogether"!

As the man sat down, the Mayor noticed this rather bulky lady seating visibly in a lateral seat, wearing a very colourful T-shirt. He pointed it to the last speaker, in an eloquent gesture. The T-Shirt red:

"Behold the turtle; He only makes progress when he sticks his neck out" [41].

References

1. Endsley S, Kibb DC, Linares A, Colorafi K. An introduction to personal health records. Family Practice Medicine. [Serial on the Internet]. 2006 May. 13 (5). Available from: http://www.aafp.org/fpm/20060500/57anin.html. (Accessed 10 January 2008).
2. Kickbusch I. Perspectives on health governance in the 21st century. In: Marinker M, editor. Health targets in Europe: polity, progress and promise. London: BMJ Books, 2002; 206–229.
3. Sakellarides, C., Stewardship. In: Marinker M., editor. Constructive conversations about health and values. Oxford: Radcliffe Publishing, 2006.
4. Sakellarides, C. El valor de la salud e su "gobierno" en un mundo globalizado posmoderno: el encuentro de la Bella y la Bestia. *Humanitas, Humanidades Médicas.* 2003; 91–100.
5. United Nations. Expanding public space for the development of the knowledge society: report of the Ad Hoc Expert Group Meeting on Knowledge systems for development. New York: Department of Economic and Social Affairs, United Nations, 2003.
6. Koch G. Conference Board of Canada. Center for Health Care Innovation. Exploring Technologic Innovation in Health Systems. August, 2007. Available from: www.conferenceboard.ca/documents.asp?rnext = 2098. (Accessed 12 February 2008).
7. Koch G. What to endow to a country which already has everything?: Finland in transition towards the Knowledge Society. In: Stale, Pirjo, editor. Five Steps for Finland's Future. Helsinki: TEKES, 2007 (Technology Review).

8. Røste, R. Studies of innovation in the public sector: a literature review. European Commission: PUBLIN, 2003. (Innovation in the Public Sector. Public Report; D16). Available from: http://www.step.no/publin/reports/d16litteraturesurvey.pdf. (Accessed 05 January 2008).
9. Cunningham, P. Innovation in the health sector: a case study analysis. European Commission: PUBLIN, 2005. (Innovation in the Public Sector. Public Report; D19). Available from: http://www.step.no/publin/reports/d19-casestudies-health.pdf. (Accessed 15 January 2008).
10. Koch, P., Hauknes J. On innovation in the public sector. European Commission: PUBLIN, 2005. (Innovation in the Public Sector. Public Report; D20). Available from: http://www.step.no/publin/reports/d20-innovation.pdf. (Accessed 18 January 2008).
11. Bacon N, et al. Transformers: how local areas innovate to address changing social needs: research report. London: NESTA – National Endowment for Science, Technology and the Arts. January 2008.
12. Chesbrough, H. Open innovation: the new imperative for creating and profiting from technology. Harvard: Harvard Business School Press, 2003.
13. Von Hippel, E. Democratizing innovation. Chap. X. Cambridge, MA: MIT Press, 2005.
14. Pratt W, Unruh, K., Civan, A. Skeels, M.M. Personal health information management. Communications of the ACM, 2006 January; 49 (1): 51–55.
15. Working Group on Policies for Electronic Information Sharing between Doctors and Patients. Connecting Americans to their healthcare: final report. New York: The Markle Foundation, 2004.
16. National Health Service. About NHSDirect. Available from: www.nhsdirect.nhs.uk. (Accessed 12 February 2008).
17. Strecher V. Internet methods for delivering behavioral and health-related interventions (eHealth). Annual Review Clinic Psychology. [Serial on the Internet]. 2007; 3: 53–76. Available from: http://clinpsy.nnualreviews.org. (Accessed 25 October 2007).
18. Pyper C. et al. Patients' experiences when accessing their on-line electronic patient records in primary care. British Journal of General Practice, 2004 January, 54 (498): 38–43.
19. Richards T. My illness, my record. British Medical Journal, 2007 March; 10.334 (7592): 510.
20. Elliot R. Siegel et al. Information Rx: Evaluation of a new informatics tool for physicians, patients, and libraries. Information Services and Use, 2006; 26(1): 1–10.
21. Personalised Information Platform for Life & Health Services. About PIPS. Available from: http://www.pips.eu.org/index.html. (Accessed 25 October 2007).
22. Marchionini G, Rimer BK, Wildemuth B. Evidence base for personal health record usability: final report to the National Cancer Institute. Chapel Hill, NC: University of North Carolina, 2007. Available from: http://www.ils.unc.edu/phr/presentations.html. (Accessed 25 November 2007).
23. The Markle Foundation. Connecting for Health. The Personal Health Working Group: Final Report. New York: The Markle Foundation, 2005. Available from: http://www.markle.org/downloadable assets/final phwg report1.pdf. (Accessed 25 November 2007).
24. AHIMA Personal Health Records Council. Helping consumers select PHRs: questions and considerations for navigating an emergent market. Journal of AHIMA, 2006 November–December; 77(10): 50–56.
25. Pagliari C, Detmer D, Singleton P. Potential of electronic health records. British Medical Journal, 2007 August; 335: 330–333.
26. National Committee on Vital and Health Statistics. Personal health records and personal health records systems. Washington, DC: US Department of Health and Human Services, 2006.
27. Pagliari C, Detmer D, Singleton P. Electronic personal health records: emergence and implications for the UK. London: The Nuffield Trust, 2007.
28. Tang PC., Ash JS, Bates DW, Overhage JM, Sands DZ. Personal Health Records: definition, benefits, and strategies for overcoming barriers to adoption. Journal of the American Medical Informatics Association, 2006 Mar–Apr; 13(2): 121–126.
29. KatrinaHealth. About Katrina Health. Available from: http://www.katrinahealth.org. (Accessed 15 January 2008).

30. Health and Human Services. About Department of Health and Human Services. Available from: http://www.hhs.gov/. (Accessed 15 January 2008).
31. Saranummi, N. Citizen-centric value network of professionals: well-being services @ work. 10 March 2004. Proc. E-Challenges E-2004, October 2004.
32. Etheredge, LM. What would a rapid-learning health system look like, and how might we get there?, A Rapid-Learning Health System. Project HOPE. Health Affairs, Maryland, 2007.
33. World Health Organization. Bridging the "Know-do" Gap Meeting on Knowledge Translation in Global Health. Geneva: WHO, 2006.
34. Multi-Organizational Partnerships, Alliances and Networks. Engagement. In: Gould N, editor. United Kingdom: University of Glamorgan, 2005.
35. Coleman S, Gotze J. Bowling together: online public engagement in policy deliberation. London: Hansard Society, 2001.
36. Morton Warner chapter.
37. The Markle Foundation. Connecting for Health. Survey finds Attitudes of Americans Regarding Personal Health Records and Nationwide Electronic Health Information Exchange. New York: The Markle Foundation, 2005. Available from: http://www.phrconference.org/assets/research_release_101105.pdf. (Accessed 10 January 2008).
38. Coulter A, Magee, H., ed. lit. The European patient of the future. Buckingham, UK: Open University Press, 2003.
39. Tapscott D, Williams A, Pinho JA, trad. Wikinomics – A nova Economia das Multidões Inteligentes. Matosinhos, Portugal: QUIDNOVI, September 2007.
40. Mandl KD, Kohane IS. Tectonic shifts in the health information economy. The New England journal of medicine. April 2008; 358 (16): 1732–1737.
41. Magretta J. What management is: How it works and why it's everyone's business. London: Profile Books, June 2003.

Index